Text Book on Physiology of Lactation

About the Authors

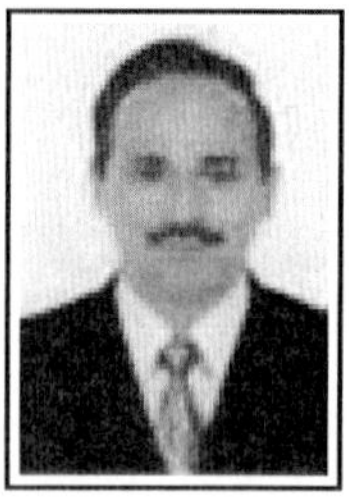

Dr. Mahendra Singh has been actively engaged in the research and teaching programme in Animal Physiology Division of the National Dairy Research Institute, Karnal since 1984. Dr. Singh main research work are lactation physiology and milk production management. Dr. Singh has been decorated with many prestigious awards for research excellence like Dr. D. Sunderesan Award, Dr. S.N. Mullick Award, Dr. P.K. Dwarka Nath Award. He has published more than 130 research publications in high rated International and National journals of repute, authored many books and acquired advance training in Dairy Science Department, University of Florida, USA. Dr. Singh has guided more than 20 MVSc and PhD students. He has been on expert panel of many scientific committees, General Secretary of the Alumni association and of Society of Animal Physiologist of India. Dr. Singh has been the officer Incharge of Cattle Yard Section and is presently working as Head- Division of Animal Physiology at ICAR-National Dairy Research Institute, Karnal.

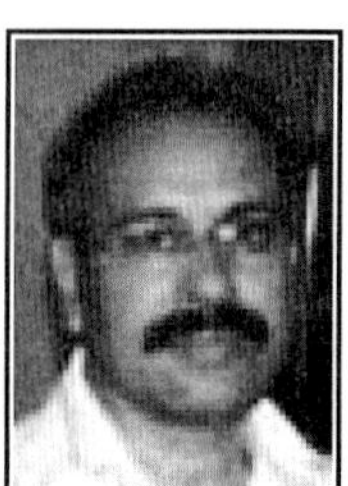

Dr A.K. Roy has been teaching the graduate and postgraduate students at National Dairy Research Institute Karnal for the last 6 years. He has been working as ARS scientist since 1985. He has also served as Professor (Veterinary Physiology) at Gondar University Ethiopia. He has published many research and popular articles in the reputed journals.

Text Book on
Physiology of Lactation

Mahendra Singh
Principal Scientist & Head
Animal Physiology Division
ICAR - National Dairy Research Institute,
Karnal-132001, HR, India (Chhokar.ms@gmail.com)

A.K. Roy
Senior Scientist (Animal Physiology)
ICAR-NDRI, Karnal
Email : royashwani@gmail.com

SSPH

SATISH SERIAL PUBLISHING HOUSE
403, Express Tower, Commercial Complex
Azadpur, Delhi-110033 (India)
Phone : 011-47073040, Fax : 91-11-27672046
e-mail : info@satishserial.com, hkjain1975@yahoo.com
Website : www.satishserial.com

Published by :

SATISH SERIAL PUBLISHING HOUSE
403, Express Tower, Commercial Complex, Azadpur, Delhi-110033 (INDIA)
Phone : 011 – 47073040 Fax : 91-11-27672046
E-mail : info@satishserial.com, hkjain1975@yahoo.com

Print Again, 2024

ISBN 978-93-86200-18-1

Composed, Designed & Printed in India

Preface

Man has been rearing many animal species for his survival and sustenance since long. Cattle, buffaloes and goats are mostly reared for milk or meat in many countries around the world. Every species has its physiology, genetic potential and production capabilities. Physiology is one of the most fascinating subjects dealing with the functions of animal body. We have got a sizable population of lactating animals in our country but the average milk production per animal is much less. While there has been a consistent growth in the production of milk horizontally over the years but the time has come to boost the same vertically. Tremendous breakthroughs have come up in the field of feeding and management of lactating animals in the recent years but we need to understand the physiological mechanisms of lactation behind milk production. There are many reference books and publications on the subject from various authors but the students of lactation physiology find difficult to grasp this subject.

The present book has been written to make the subject easy to understand while highlighting the latest advances in the subject of lactation. The book has not only discussed the basic structure, functioning of mammary gland and practical aspects of increasing milk production but also explained the lactation physiology in the simplest language. We hope that this book will be useful for the students of animal husbandry and veterinary degree students at UG and PG levels. We have no doubt that the publication will not only cater to the needs of graduates and postgraduate students studying the lactation physiology but also meet the requirements of animal enthusiasts in our country.

Authors

Contents

Chapter-1

Selection of a Good Dairy Animal

To begin with the dairy farming, selection of a good animal is prerequisite for success and better income. The ability of the animal to secrete milk depends upon the genetic constitution of the animal. Therefore, dairy animals with high milk yield, longer lactation length, shorter inter-calving period and adequate disease resistance should be selected. Some of the important points for selecting a good dairy animal are listed below.

- The animal can be selected on the basis of shape of horns for characterization and identification of a specific breed.
- Animal should be free from any disease and external abnormalities.
- Body condition of the animals should be sound (score 4-5). The body condition score also indicates energy status of the animal.
- The body of lactating cow or buffalo should not be too lean or too fatty.
- Udder of the animal should be well developed, balanced and should have firm attachments to the body without any visual deformity.
- The milk vein should be prominent as it has been reported to be an important index of milk producing ability of the animal.
- Animal with large udder should be selected as they have more amount of glandular or milk secreting tissue which can be felt by hand palpation. Smaller mammary glands have little udder capacity and unable to secrete and store more milk.
- Teats should be of normal size and free from abrasion, leakage of milk or any other external deformity.
- For efficient machine milking, short and thinner teats are good. Also the direction of teats and their proper placement is essential which ensures proper attachment of teat-cups and prevents falling

of milk claw during machine milking. Very small teats are undesirable for the hand and machine milking operations.

- Milch animals should possess docile type of milking temperament. Animals showing aggressive behaviour consume more time and may harm the milkman or damage the machines at the time of milking. Such animals also produce less milk and may have shorter lactation period.
- The lactating animal should not be a repeat breeder or should not have any kind of reproductive health problem which makes them unfit for the normal reproduction process.
- Lactating animals should have an inter-calving period of 12-14 months in order to make dairying a profitable business.
- The subcutaneous fat should not be more; as such cow or buffalo has a tendency to get obese with good feeding management whereas the effect on milk yield is much less.
- Animal should be free from any infectious disease, should be apparently healthy.
- The skin coat should have luster/shining.

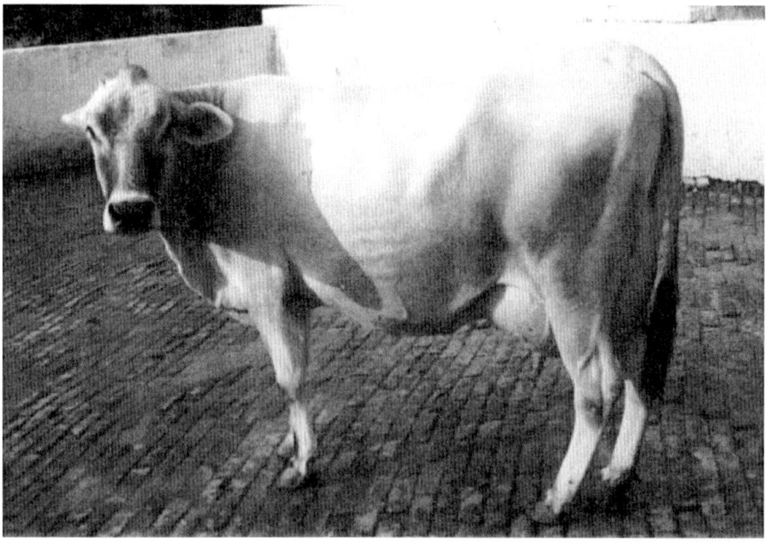

Photo: A healthy lactating crossbred cow

❑❑❑

Chapter-2

Milk Composition

Milk is defined as the whole, fresh, clean, lacteal secretion of the mammary gland which can be obtained by complete milking of healthy milch animals and contains the minimum prescribed percentage of milk fat and milk solids not fat (SNF). It is also known as the nutritive fluid for the infants. The price of milk is usually determined by its fat and or SNF content.

Colostrum: Colostrum is the first lacteal secretion of the mammary gland obtained after the calving and is present up to 6 milking. It is essential for the newborn calf to receive colostrum within the first 36 hours of birth. If cow is not producing colostrum due to some reason, colostrum of another cow or from artificial sources should be fed to the newborn. It contains antibodies, growth factors and is superior in nutritional value as compared to milk. Colostrum provides passive immunity to disease and helps to build up vitamin and mineral levels. Once the calf has received colostrum, it can be fed solely on whole milk or milk replacers.

At birth a calf's immune system is not fully developed. Colostrum imparts passive immunity from the dam to the newborn calf via intestinal absorption of antibodies. Therefore, it should be fed for the first 3 days after birth. The quality and volume of the colostrum produced by a cow depends on her lactation number and breed. Vitamins like A, D and E do not cross the placenta from the cow to the calf. Thus calves are born with low levels of vitamins and are dependent on adequate consumption of good quality colostrum to boost initial levels of these vitamins. Colostrum usually contains 6-10 times more of vitamin D than that of ordinary milk. Inadequate feeding, or quality of colostrum is a primary cause of low immunity in calves.

A successful colostrum management program requires farmers to consistently provide calves with a sufficient volume of clean, high-quality colostrum within the first few hours of life. As time from birth increases the ability of the calf to absorb the antibodies is reduced.

Absorption is greatest in the first few hours of life and starts to decline progressively after 4 to 6 hours and ceases after 24 hours from birth. Therefore, it is critical to feed colostrum as soon as possible after calving to ensure maximum immunity. It should also be noted that there is evidence to suggest that the concentration of antibodies in colostrum decreases by 3.7 % per hour from calving.

Milk plasma is defined as milk minus the milk fat globules, which is close in composition to skim milk (or separated milk) although the separation of fat from rest of the milk is never complete.

Milk serum is defined as milk plasma minus casein micelles, which is close to the composition of whey, except for the presence of some of the proteolytic products from chymosin.

Table. Composition of milk in different species

Species	Percentage of Composition				
	Water	Fat	Protein	Lactose	Ash
Ass	90.0	1.3	1.7	6.5	0.5
Buffalo	84.2	6.6	3.9	5.2	0.8
Camel	86.5	3.1	4.0	5.6	0.8
Cat	84.6	3.8	9.1	4.9	0.6
Cow	86.6	4.6	3.4	4.9	0.7
Dog	75.4	9.6	11.2	3.1	0.7
Elephant	67.8	19.6	3.1	8.8	0.7
Ewe	79.4	8.6	6.7	4.3	1.0
Goat	86.5	4.5	3.5	4.7	0.8
Guinea pig	82.2	5.5	8.5	2.9	0.9
Human	87.7	3.6	1.8	6.8	0.1
Llama	86.5	3.2	3.9	5.6	0.8
Mare	89.1	1.6	2.7	6.1	0.5
Porpoise	41.1	45.8	11.2	1.3	0.6
Reindeer	68.2	17.1	10.4	2.3	1.5
Sow	89.6	4.8	1.3	3.4	0.9
Whale	70.1	19.6	9.5	–	1.0

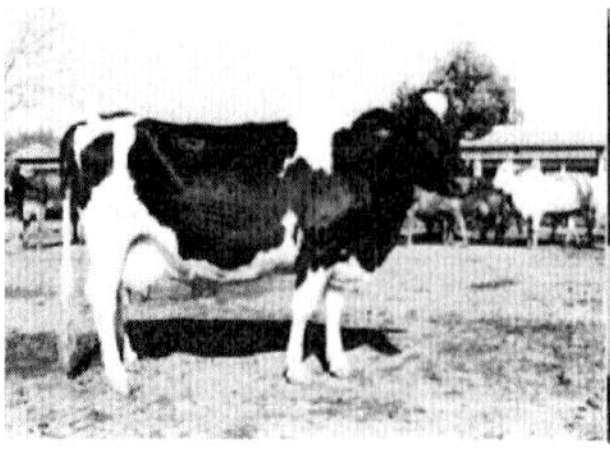
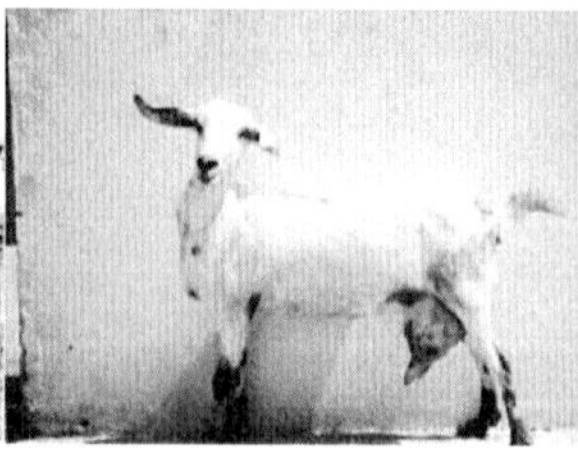
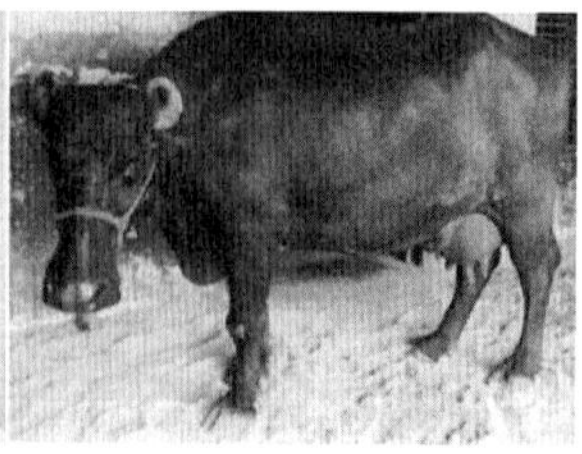

Table. Chemical composition of milk in different breeds of cow and Murrah buffalo

Species	Percentage of Composition				
	Water	**Fat**	**Protein**	**Lactose**	**Ash**
Cow Holstein	87.74	3.40	3.22	4.87	0.68
Shorthorn	87.19	3.94	3.32	4.99	0.70
Ayreshire	87.10	4.00	3.58	4.67	0.68
BrownSwiss	86.59	4.01	3.61	5.04	0.73
Guernsey	85.39	4.95	3.91	4.93	0.74
Jersey	85.09	5.37	3.92	4.93	0.71
Sindhi	86.07	4.90	3.42	4.91	0.70
Gir	86.44	4.73	3.32	4.85	0.66
Tharparkar	86.58	4.55	3.36	4.83	0.68
Sahiwal	86.42	4.55	3.33	5.04	0.66
Buffalo Murrah	83.63	6.56	3.88	5.23	0.70

(*Source:* www.dairyforall.com)

Milk composition: Milk usually contains water, carbohydrate (lactose), fat, protein, minerals, vitamins and enzymes. The composition of milk varies from species to species and within breeds. Milk composition is affected by the dietary intake, climatic conditions, management of animals, disease and is different during different stages of lactation. Milk is secreted as a complex mixture of these compounds.

Carbohydrate

Lactose is the major carbohydrate in the milk of most species. Lactose is a disaccharide composed of monsaccharides, D glucose and D-galactose, joined in a β-1, 4-glycosidic linkage. The chemical name for the lactose (milk sugar) is 4-o-β-D-galactopyranosyl-D-glucopyranose. Lactose has also been identified in the fruits of certain plants.

Role of lactose: Lactose plays a major role in the milk synthesis. It is the major osmole in milk. The process of synthesis of lactose is responsible for drawing water into the milk as it is being formed in the mammary epithelial cells. Because of the close relationship between lactose synthesis and the amount of water drawn into milk, lactose content is the least variable component of milk. The carbohydrates other than lactose are present in very low concentrations (glucose-about 0.1mM) and free galactose (about 0.2 mM). Milk which is produced under organic farming system (organic milk) is higher in omega 3-fatty acids, vitamin A, β-carotene, vitamin E and certain other antioxidants than non-organic milk. Organic milk comes from cows that graze on pastures which are not sprayed with synthetic chemical pesticides. The organic milk is usually treated gently during the whole process from milking to the subsequent processing.

Protein: The concentration of protein affects moisture, texture, flavour and yield of milk cheese. The proteins are found in the form of casein (75-85%), β-lactoglobulin (7-12%) and α-lactalbumin (2-5%) in the milk. The nitrogen content of milk is multiplied by a factor of 6.38 (15% nitrogen in proteins) to calculate total proteins in milk while non-protein nitrogen, NPN range from 2 to 10% of the "total proteins." It is not easier to change the protein content of milk because dietary nitrogen going to milk protein is low (25-30%). Over 90% of the proteins in milk are made in the udder from amino acids, glucose and acetate. The rumen microbes provide 50-75% of the amino acids while rumen un-degradable proteins provide the rest. Milk proteins are higher during the first month, decline at peak and increase after 250 days of lactation. Milk proteins vary due to breed, genetic merit, stage of lactation, season and udder health status.

Fat: Milk fat contains approximately 3.4% total fat. Over 400 individual fatty acids have been identified in milk fat. However, approximately 15 to 20 fatty acids make up 90% of the milk fat. Milk have major saturated fatty acids bearing 4 to 18 carbons (4:0, 6:0, 8:0, 10:0, 12:0, 14:0, 16:0, 18:0), monounsaturated fatty acids (16:1, 18:1), and polyunsaturated fatty acids (18:2, 18:3). Some of the fatty acids are found in very small amounts but contribute to the unique and desirable flavor of milk fat and butter. For example, the C14:0 and C16:0 ß-hydroxy fatty acids spontaneously form lactones upon heating which enhance the flavor of butter.

Minerals and vitamins: Milk is a good source of calcium, magnesium, phosphorus, potassium, selenium, and zinc. Many minerals in milk are in the form of salts, such as calcium phosphate. In milk approximately 67% of the calcium, 35% of the magnesium, and 44% of the phosphate are salts bound within the casein micelle and the remainder are soluble in the serum phase. Milk contains small amounts of copper, iron, manganese, and sodium. Milk contains the water soluble vitamins thiamin (vitamin B_1), riboflavin (vitamin B_2), niacin (vitamin B_3), pantothenic acid (vitamin B_5), vitamin B_6 (pyridoxine), vitamin B_{12} (cobalamin), vitamin C, and folate. Milk is a good source of thiamin, riboflavin and vitamin B_{12}. Milk contains the fat soluble vitamins A, D, E, and K.

❑❑❑

Chapter-3

Factors Affecting Milk Yield and Composition

The yield of milk and its chemical composition strongly influence profitability of dairy farming, therefore it is essential that udder of a cow should be free from any infection.The composition of milk is mainly influenced by nutrition, climate and health of animal. Beside this other non-nutritional factor like stage of lactation, parity, age and mastitis also influence composition of milk.

Age of the animal

Milk composition changes with an increase in the age of animals. Although fat and protein contents decrease with increasing age but these changes are small and non-significant. Since animals are often maintained upto 4 or 5 lactations and replaced later with the young stock or heifers; the age composition of the herd is unlikely to contribute significantly to variation in milk composition.

Parity

Increasing number of lactation (parity) affects milk composition. First calvers have low milk yield which increases with growing parity. Milk yield increases with an increase in the number of calving (parity) till 5th lactation and thereafter declines.

Stage of lactation

Milk yield and composition change during different stages of lactation. After the parturition, milk yield increases steadily and the peak is attained by the animal between 25 to 90 days (av. 45 days). During this time the fat and protein composition remain almost same; however once lactation is established, the protein and fat percentage increase after 90-100 days of lactation. During late lactation, milk yield decrease and fat (%) increase due to effect of pregnancy.The milk yield decline during later part of lactation whereas milk fat, sodium and chloride contents increase due to the effect of pregnancy.

Pregnancy

Early stages of pregnancy do not affect composition and yield of milk. The effects of pregnancy on milk yield and composition are visible during mid pregnancy onwards. With the advancement of pregnancy the milk yield decreases and the fat percentage increases. The concentration of sodium and chloride also increase in milk and the taste of milk becomes salty.

Climate and season

Climate affects metabolism of the lactating cows and buffaloes by influencing feed intake, changes in hormones of lactation and metabolism. High ambient temperature during summer (May-August) decreases feed intake; reduces milk yield (10-20 %) and alters milk composition. Lactating animals are more vulnerable to heat stress (high temperature) than the cold stress (low ambient temperature). To alleviate the effect of high temperature animal should be given *ad lib* water to drink. Use of ceiling fans also improves feed intake and milk production (10-15%) in summer (Figure). During extreme cold temperature ($< 8^0C$) animals should be kept in-houses and windows should be covered with gunny bags. Paddy straw bedding (6-8 inches) on floor could be used for comfort and warmth to the animal body. Season of the year has a profound effect on milk yield and composition. Cows that calve in summer months have low milk yield and low fat contents in comparison to cows that calve in the winter months. The effect of season on milk yield is mainly influenced by the quality and quantity of feed. During summer season, the poor quality of green fodder and high ambient temperature-humidity adversely affects quality of milk. The milk somatic cell counts (SCC) which is an index of the udder health and quality of milk also increase during summer season and decline during winter season.

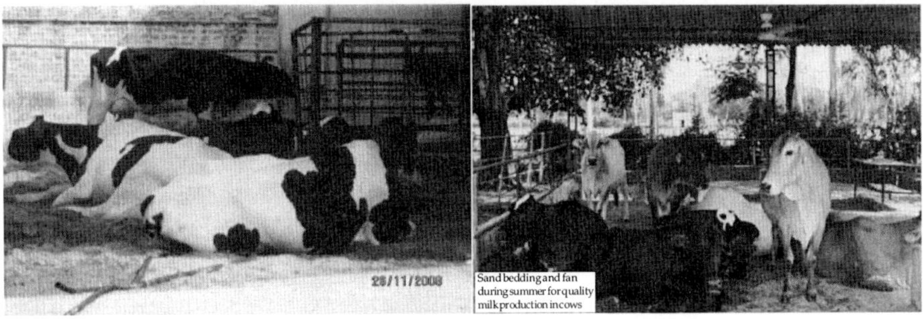
28/11/2008
Sand bedding and fan during summer for quality milk production in cows

Fig. Sand bedding and fan provides more comfort to cows in summer season

Nutrition

Nutrition is one of the most important rate limiting factor in the milk secretion of dairy animals. It affects not only the body condition of the cows and buffaloes, but also yield and composition of the milk. The crude fibre content of the roughage should be > 17-18 % in the diet of a lactating animal. In case of less CF contents, as happen during the summer season, there is a drop in the milk fat which is known as *Low milk fat syndrome*. In order to maintain the normal fat content of milk, dairy animals should be provided with sufficient crude fiber in the diet so that acetate production in the rumen is not affected. Providing supplementary feed in the form of cereal grain or concentrate mixture usually results in increased milk and protein yields. An increase in milk yield causes a decrease in fat yield. Therefore animals need to be given adequate concentrate mixture based on milk yield during lactation. When concentrates are fed, the degree of processing can affect the fat percentage of the milk. The concentrate mixture should be palatable, and grounded for better intake and digestibility. Over-processing of grains can reduce the fat percentage of the milk. Considerable research has been carried out on the the effect of protein and energy supplementation on milk yield of cows and buffaloes. Lactating animals generally use protein supplements as a source of energy rather than a supply of protein to the udder. Feeding of protein supplements increases the energy content of the total diet, as a result the protein percentage of the milk is increased.

It has been found that energy restriction in the ration of a cow decreases BCS, milk yield, plasma glucose, insulin and insulin-like growth factor-I whereas BHBA, plasma urea nitrogen and growth hormone concentration increases in cows fed a low energy (25% concentrate) as compared to a high energy (75% concentrate) diet in early lactation. While the nature of the signalling pathway(s) which links milk production to nutritional status is unknown, restricted energy intake has been shown to decrease mammary blood flow and uptake of nutrients for milk production witout influencing mammary tissue regression via apoptosis. However, active secretory cells may enter a quiescent non-secretory state and may die via apoptosis. The cells can be reactivated to restore normal milk yield when energy level of the diet improves.

Ferquency of milking

In a routine practice the dairy cows are milked twice daily. However in intensive dairying system with high yielding cows (>15 kg/d) , the milking frequency can be increased between 3 and 6 times/ day to increase milk production and relieve the udder of high milk pressure. Once-a day milking is practiced in cows and buffaloes when the yield become very less. Some researchers have pointed out reduced milk yield (22%), lactation length and persistency of lactation with once a day milking practice in cows. At the same time beneficial effects of once a day milking are better farm management, reduced labor requirements, less expenditures, better health, faster postpartum metabolic adjustments in negative energy balance (NEBAL) during early lactation and in lean season of the fodder.

Table. Milk Yield and component responses to twice daily (2x) vs. three times daily (3x) milking frequency for primiparous and multiparous cows (Erdman *et al.*, 1995).

Parity	Milking Frequency	Milk Yield (kg/day)	Fat%	Fat Yield (g/day)
Primiparous	2x	18.7	3.69	769
	3x	22.0	3.62	859
Multiparous(>one calf)	2x	19.1	3.65	894
	3x	22.6	3.48	987
Difference (3X-2X)	3.5	-0.17	93	

Reduced milking frequencies significantly slow down the milk secreted by the mammary cells and could result in the production loss of 29%-33% as compared to 2x milking during the previous lactation. Increases in milk production by 8-10% for 3x and 12-16% for 4x and 21% from 3x to 6x have been observed in many studies. The increased milk yields were due to increased secretory cell numbers and higher prolactin hormone being secreted at each milking in early lactation. It also improves persistency of lactation. Several studies have indicated that primiparous cows respond better during 3 to 4x milking due to their smaller udder capacity. The other reasons of increase in milk yield with increased milking frequency are due to :

- Increased cell number
- Decreased apoptosis
- Availability of more nutrients to the mammary gland
- Less intramammary pressure in the mammary gland

Effect on milk composition and metabolism

Milk composition and quality is either unchanged or improved by more frequent milking relative to 2x. Reduction in milking frequency from 2x to 1x result in increase in protein, fat, serum albumin, sodium, chloride and SCC, but a decrease in the concentrations of lactose and potassium. However, an increased milking frequency in early lactation may create a greater state of NEBAL due to the increased mobilisation of body reserves and inadequate feed intake to support milk synthesis.

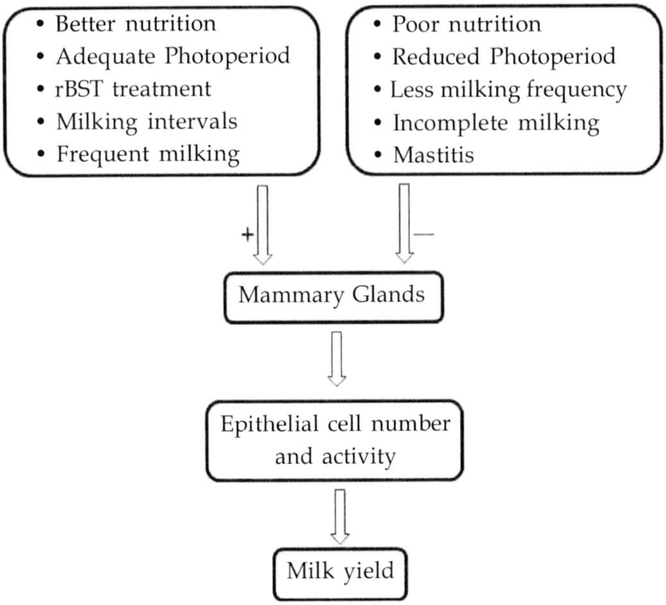

Factors affecting milk yield in dairy animals

❒❒❒

Chapter-4

Structure of Udder

External structure of udder

Mammary gland is an apocrine gland i.e. intermediate between exocrine and holocrine. It secretes milk along with small amount of cellular debris. Mammary Gland is located in inguinal region in cattle, buffalo, sheep, mare and goat. In cows and buffaloes, four mammary glands combine to form a structure known as *Udder*, while in goats two mammary glands (quarter) form the udder. All the four mammary glands of udder are separated from each other internally and synthesize milk independently. The shape of udder is generally cylindrical or oval (Figure 1 a Jersey cow). In Mare, blood and lymph systems are similar to the cow's. However, Mare has two flat but broad blunt teats with each teat having two streak canals and two cisterns. Each cistern joins a separate gland. Therefore mare also has 4 "quarters" like a cow but 2 streak canals per teat like a Pig. Pig has the charactieristic of having 12-14 glands (6-7 pair) which may also be upto 6-32. These mammary glands are independent and could be paired or unpaired. A healthy udder of a lactating animal is very soft on palpitations by hand and is indicative of more parenchyma tissue which synthesizes milk, while hard udder indicates less parenchyma. Any external injury or increase in the size of udder indicate likely incidence of udder inflammation or mastitis disease. Pain in the udder by hand touch indicates infection or inflammation in the mammary gland. Udder remains attached to the body by strong median suspensory ligament which divides the udder into right and left part (Figure). But further division of right and left part is not easily distinguishable from the exterior.

A good dairy animal has a large and prominent mammary vein also called milk vein. High producing animals could be characterized by a large and well developed udder which is firmly attached with the body (Figure 2). Mammary gland of the dairy animal is independent of each other and drains milk with an independent teat. Milk which is synthesized in one gland (*also called quarter*) cannot pass over to any of the other gland or quarter. The right and left side of udder are separated externally by a distinct median suspensory ligament. Numerous lamellae (branches) extend from this ligament into the quarters to provide support to the udder. Front and hind quarters are more diffusely separated and cannot be differentiated externally. Internally all the four quarters of a cow udder are independent of each other from the functional point of view. Each quarter is made up of secretory tissue (*alveoli*), ducts, gland and teat cistern which store milk. The teat canal and teat drain out milk during milking. Milk synthesis and secretion is a continuous process and filling of udder with milk between milking stretches the udder like a balloon. Udder is also covered with fine hairs and the density of hair varies in different species.

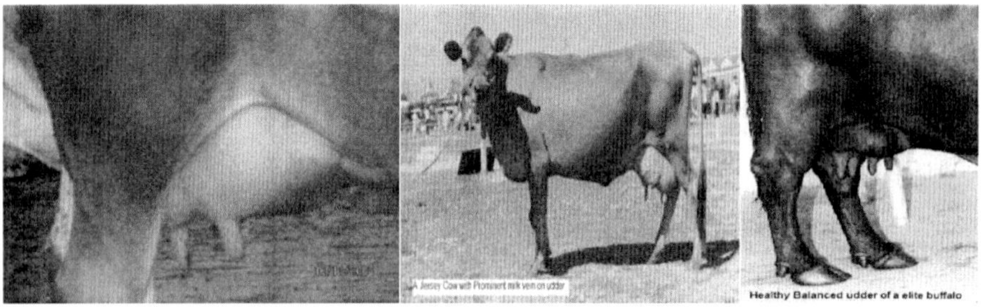

Figure 1. A healthy udder of a cow and buffalo

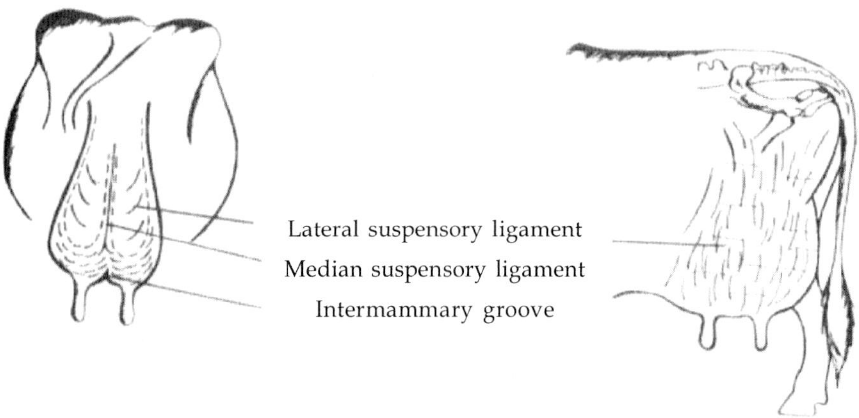

Figure 2. External structure of udder

Teats

Each quarter of udder has one teat to drain out the milk. Thus four teats are present in cows and buffaloes. In addition to the four teats, cows may have some additional teats called supernumerary teats or extra teats. These teats may be located on lateral side, intercalary position, anterior or posterior position. These teats are not used for milking but may cause infection in the udder. Therefore, they should be removed in growing stage of calf. Udder may have hairs on its surface but teat lack hair. The skin of teat is provided with sensory nerves which are sensitive to calf suckling and hand milking stimulus.

Score	Description	Illustration
N	**No ring** The teat-end is smooth with a small, even orifice. This is a typical status for many teats soon after the start of lactation	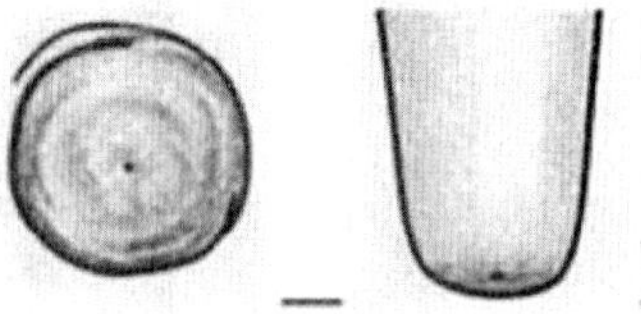
S	**Smooth or Slightly rough ring** A raised ring encircles the office. The surface of the ring is smooth or it may feel slightly rough but no fronds of old keratin are evident.	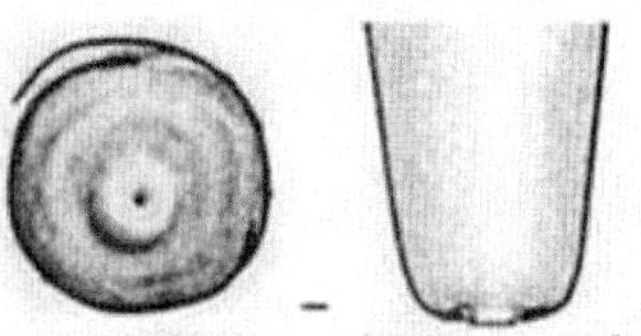
R	**Rough ring** A raised, roughened ring with isolated fronds or mounds of old keratin extending 1 - 3 mm from the orifice.	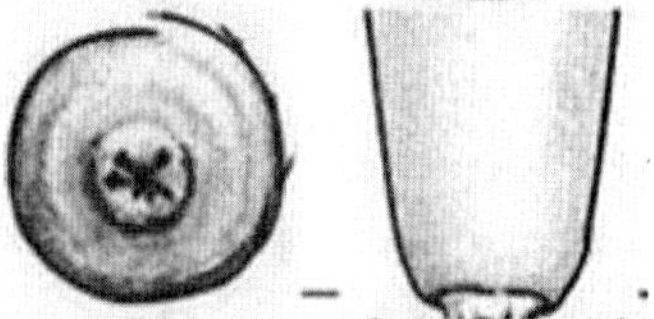
VR	**Very Rough ring** A raised ring with rough fronds or mounds of old keratin extending 4 mm or more the orifice. The rim of the ring is rough and cracked, often giving the teat-end a "flowered" appearance.	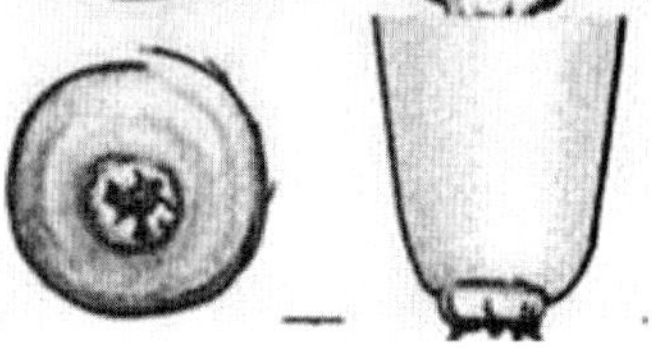

Teat score with R and VR are not suitable for machine milking

Each teat of a quarter opens internally into teat cistern and a teat canal. At the junction of teat cistern and teat canal, a Fursternberg's rosette made up of 6-10 longitudinal folds is present. This rosette has got a physiological significance that- i) it prevents entry of pathogens into the udder, ii) provides local defence against mastitis causing pathogen and iii) smooth muscles of teat canal remain closed between two milkings. The teat canal is also provided with Keratin or Keratin like substances which act as an effective barrier for the entry of harmful bacteria. At the end of teat, the teat pore is present to drain out the milk. This pore remains closed between milking by a circular sphincter muscle called teat sphincter near the tip. Teat sphincter muscles i) prevent entry of pathogens (bacteria) and ii) effectively check oozing out of milk against the gravity force. The skin of teat is provided with nerve fibres and nerve endings which are sensitive to the suckling stimulus, hand and machine milking stimulus. The teat skin is also sensitive to heat and cold stimuli.

Internal Structure

Udder is made up of pink and white tissue. The pink color tissue is called parenchyma or epithelial tissue while white tissue or non-parenchyma cells are made up of connective, fibrous and fatty tissue. Internal structure of udder has following parts.

Teat Pore – It is the small opening at the end of teat which drains out the milk during milking. It remains tightly closed by teat sphincter muscle. Teat sphincter muscles do not allow leakage of milk between milkings (Figure 3).

Teat Canal – It is a narrow canal which lies within the teat and opens in the teat cistern. At the junction of teat canal and teat cistern, special folds are present which prevent flow of milk against gravity force. These folds are called Furstenberg's Rosettes. The teat canal is an important barrier against entry of microorganism into the udder. The teat canal is 8 -12 mm in length and can store 15 to 40 ml of milk, depending on the size of the teat. Cows with small teat canal or tight sphincter muscle take more time in milking and are refered to as slow milkers. Animals with large teat canal or weak sphincter muscle suffer from leakage of milk from teats between milking and are more prone to mastitis-causing organisms. Udder is also provided with nerves connected to the smooth muscles in the circulatory system and the smooth muscles in the milk ducts.

Gland Cistern- Each teat has one cistern which stores milk (400-500 ml) between the milkings. Gland cistern is located just above the teat cistern and is partially separated by annular folds of tissue.

Large Ducts and Small Ducts- Small ducts open into the large milk ducts which then carry milk into the gland cistern. The small ducts carry the milk synthesized by each alveolus. The ductal system of the udder consists of many larger and smaller ducts in the order of;

1. Lobar ducts, 2. Intra-lobar duct 3. Inter-loubular duct and 4. Intralobular ducts. The main function of the duct system is to;

i) Collect milk from the secretory tissue

ii) Store a part of the milk between milkings and

iii) Transport the milk into the gland cistern

Large and small ducts have constrictions at the point of each branch of duct to prevent drain of milk and leaking into the teat.

Lobes and Lobules - Each mammary gland is made up of numerous lobes. Each lobe is made up of many lobules. Lobes and lobules are separated by connective tissue layers. Each lobule contains up to 200-250 alveoli. Each alveolus is made up of single layer of epithelial cells.

Epithelial cells – These cells synthesize milk and secrete the milk into lumen of alveoli.

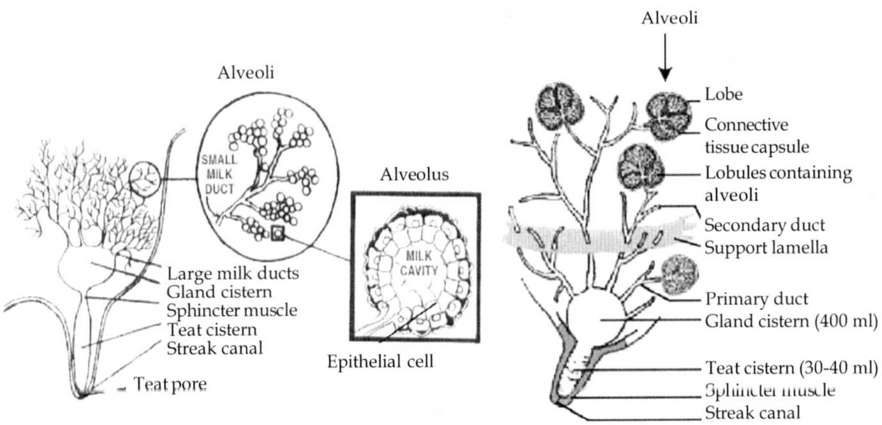

Figure 3. Internal structure of udder

The functional milk-producing unit of udder is the alveolus which is spherical in shape. The outer surface of alveolus is lined with a single layer of epithelial cells and a small duct to drain out the milk called alveolar duct. The outer layer of alveolus also contains muscle-like cells called *myoepithelial cells*. These cells have receptors for the binding of oxytocin, a hormone essential for the let down of milk. Oxytocin binding to the receptors contracts the cell causing letdown of milk in lumen of alveoli. The contraction of myoepithelial cells can raise the intramammary pressure upto 60 mmHg or more. At this pressure the milk secretion is effectively stopped.

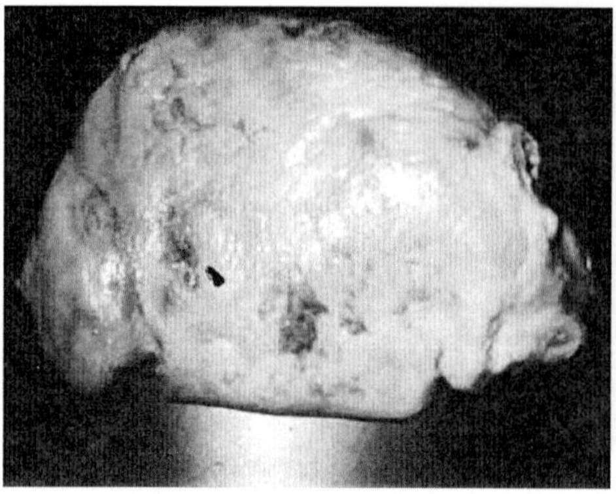

Picture of udder after removal of skin

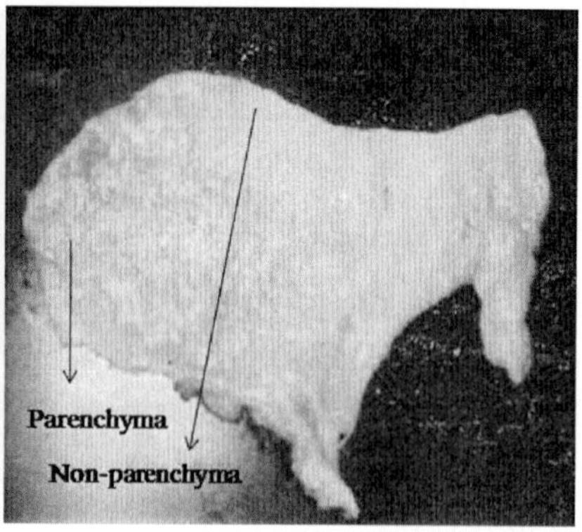

Light and dark patches indicate non-parenchyma and paraenchyma tissue

A group of alveoli form a lobule and a group of lobules, in turn, forms the main lobe of each quarter. The udder of the dairy cow contains about 5 x 10^{12} secretory cells in the alveolar tissue. Mammary gland of a cow or buffalo consists of pink colored secretory parenchyma tissue and connective tissue which is non-parenchyma. The amount of secretory tissue or secreting cells determines the quantity of milk produced by animals. Thus parenchyma is the rate limiting factor in milk producing capacity of udder. It is a common belief that a big udder is related to a high milk production capacity however, this is not true in general. A big udder might include a lot of connective and adipose tissue which allows less space for milk-secreting tissue. Udders which shrink noticeably and become flabby after milking contain less connective tissue. The milk is synthesized in the secretory cells (epithelial cells), which are arranged as a single layer on a basal membrane in a spherical structure called alveoli. The diameter of each alveolus is about 50-250 mm. Milk which is continuously synthesized by the epithelial cells is stored in the lumen of alveoli's, larger and smaller milk ducts and the gland and teat cistern between milkings.

In an udder, about 60-80% of the milk is stored in the alveoli and small milk ducts, while cistern contains 20-40% milk. Milk which is stored in alveoli is called 'alveolar milk' while that of cistern is called 'cistern milk'. The percentage of cistern milk is more in cows than in buffaloes. Buffaloes have more alveolar milk (about 90-95 %) in comparison to cows. Due to this reason buffaloes require adequate teat message before start of milking to let down the alveolar milk into gland and teat cistern.

❑❑❑

Chapter-5

Suspensory Structure of Udder

The weight of cow's udder is around 50 kg including milk and blood, but it can weigh up to 100 kg. Being a heavy and delicate structure, it is firmly attached to the body skeleton and muscles to avoid any injury and incidence of mastitis. The main components of the suspensory udder are as follows.

1. Skin protects the udder and gives the distinct shape to it. Udder's skin attaches itself to the animal body and provides a minor support to the udder.
2. Another structure that provides minor support is the areolar subcutaneous tissue which attaches skin to the underlying tissue.
3. The coarse areolar tissue which is like a cord, attaches the dorsal part of front quarter with the wall of abdomen. It is an important supporting structure as weakening of this tissue results in the detachement of udder from the udder wall.
4. Median suspensory ligament is made up of two heavy sheets of yellow elastic fibrous tissue which divide the udder into left and right halves. It stretches as the udder fills with milk.
5. The lateral suspensory ligament attaches the lateral side of udder with the body. It is made up of fibrous connective tissue without any elasticity. It sends number of lamellae into the udder and is continuous with interstitial framework. The front and rear quarters of each half of the udder are further divided internally by a very thin wall of connective tissue which cannot be differentiated from outside. The secretory tissue is supported by web-like connective tissue which cris-crosses the udder. The median suspendory ligament provides central udder support. If this ligament is weakened then the udder becomes pendulous and teats face outwards. Such teats lead to difficult milking operations and udder becomes more susceptible to injury and contamination by dirt or bacteria.

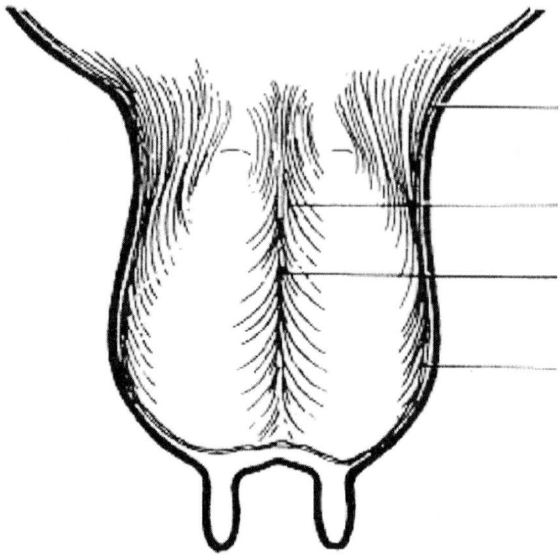

Figure. Supporting structures of a cow mammary gland

Blood supply of udder

The udder is supplied with well developed arterial and venous system. Arteries carry blood to the mammary glands for maintaining the milk synthesis. In cows and buffaloes the venous blood is carried by two routes into the heart. i) Many small veins join together in the upward direction and enter into the venous cycle to form external pudic vein which carries blood in upward direction. ii) Subcutaneous abdominal vein pours blood into the anterior vena cava after passing ventrally through diaphragm. Subcutaneous abdominal vein is also called milk vein. This vein is prominent in high producing animals. This vein enlarges just behind the ribs and forms a swollen structure called milk well. Two thirds of the venous blood passes via external pudic vein, while one third blood flows through the subcutaneous abdominal vein. However, arterial blood flows only in one direction through single route i.e. from the heart downward to mammary gland through external pudic artery.

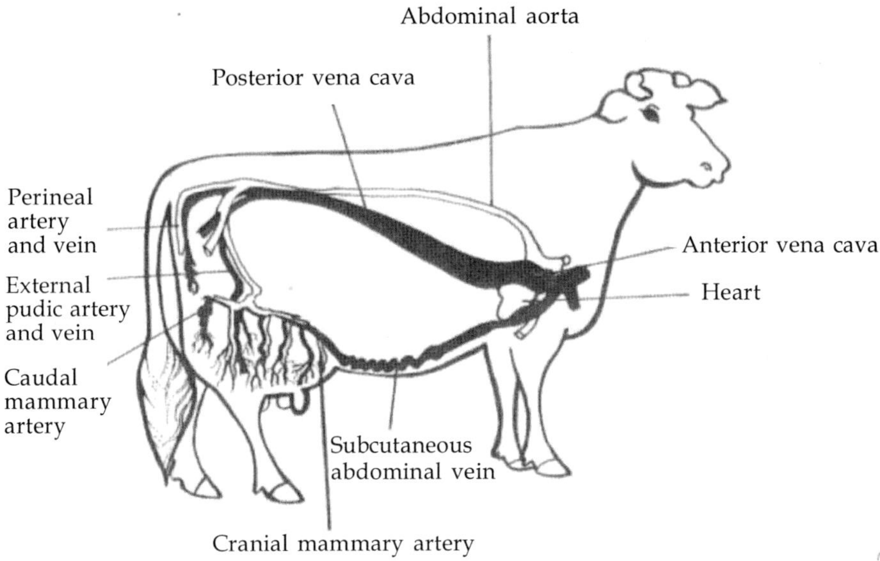

Figure. Arterial and venous system of udder

Venous Circle

During lactation about 500 litres of blood have to pass through the udder to synthesize 1 litre of milk. For a cow producing 60 litres of milk/day, 30,000 litre of blood is circulated through the mammary glands. Aorta has a blood pressure of about 140 mm which declines to 25 mm in the small capillaries of udder. The low pressure gradient leads to the driving of nutrients from blood to epithelial cells for the synthesis of milk. The teat contains many blood vessels with small valves that maintain blood flow when the teat is massaged by hand and the teat cup liner. Lack of massage during milking causes blood and other body fluids to dam-up in the teat. This is painful and causes irritation to the animal.

In addition to blood supply, udder also contains lymphatic system which carries waste products away from the udder. A pair of supramammary lymph nodes serves as a filter for foreign substances and produce lymphocytes to fight infections. The accumulation of fluids in the interstitial spaces leads to the swelling of udder called *edema*. The incidence of udder edema is more around parturition in high milk producing cows and first calvers. Udder edema is partly caused by the presence of milk in the udder which compresses the lymphatics.

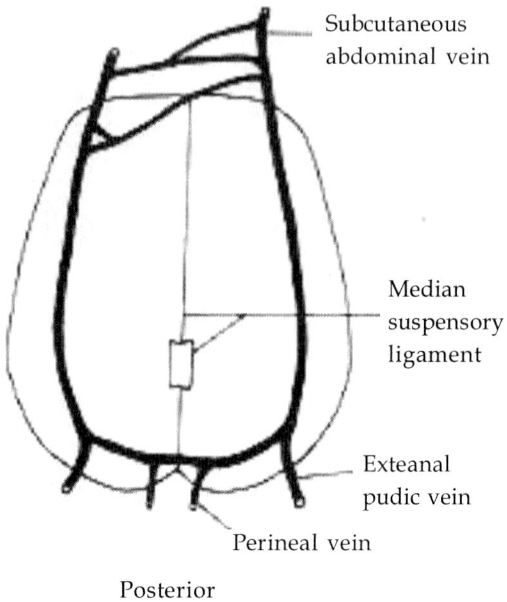

Figure. Venous circle of the udder

The venous circle has advantage of sending the blood to alternate route. When subcutaneous abdominal vein is compressed during siting of animal on floor, the venous flow of blood is maintained by the external pudic vein. In a standing animal the majority of blood to the heart is sent via subcutaneous abdormial vein.

The venous circle is formed by anastomosing of anterior and posterior mammary veins. It effectively prevents pinching off the areas of venous outflow when the cow is lying down. A lying cow also has an increased blood diffusion through the udder (around 5 L/min) compared with a standing animal (around 3L/min). This improves udder function and milk production.

Sigmoid flexure - Just below the inguinal canal, the pudic artery forms an S-shaped flexure. This allows the downward distension of udder with gradual filling of milk so that blood vessels are not stressed. Generally, there is no mixing up of blood supply between the two udder halves.

❑❑❑

Chapter-6

Role of Nervous System in Lactation

The mammary gland epithelial cells are mainly governed by the hormones for milk secretion and development. The release of hormone is controlled by nervous system. The nervous system sends appropriate signals of stress or comfort to the brain. The mammary gland is supplied with sympathetic and parasympathetic innervations.

Parasympathetic system is associated with the release of acetylcholine and includes parts of cranial and sacral nerves.

Cranial nerves are ;

3rd (occilomotor) → Control Iris function

7th (facial) → Control lacrimal or tear glands

9th (glossopharyngial) → Control salivary glands

10th (vagus) → Control heart, lungs, digestive tract & spleen

Sacral spinal nerve no. 1, 2 & 3 innervate urinary bladder, colon and external genitalia.

Sympathetic nervous system is functional when animal is frightened or fleeing. It is supplied by a number of ganglions along the sides of vertebral column, which sends signals to the periphery. Any stress that activates sympathetic innervations may lead to-

- Dilation of pupils in the eyes
- Vasoconstriction of blood vessels in the salivary glands
- Increase in heart rate (HR)
- Increased rate of blood flow to GI tract and pancreas
- Release of stress hormones like cortisol, epinephrine and norepinephrine
- Reduced blood flow to urinary bladder and mammary glands

Nerves which are supplied to the udder from the brain are the first four lumber nerves. Udder tissue has scanty nerve innervations which are mainly sympathetic fibers supplying to the arterioles. A few nerve fibers innervate walls of the ducts, cisterns and sphincter muscle of the teats. There is vasoconstriction due to the stimulation of sympathetic nervous system which causes teat contraction and reduction in the blood flow rate by creating resistance to the flow of blood. The let down of milk or increase in the udder pressure stimulate sensory nerve fibers and milking stress is generated. This kind of stress exists in most of the species. The sensory nerves are very few in the udder and the mammary tissue is insensitive to cut or pinching in some species. It has been reported that nerves are not found near the myoepithelial and epithelial cells but teats are consists of sensory or sympathetic innervations. Teat wall has free sensory nerve endings which are sensitive to pain, cold, warmth or pressure.

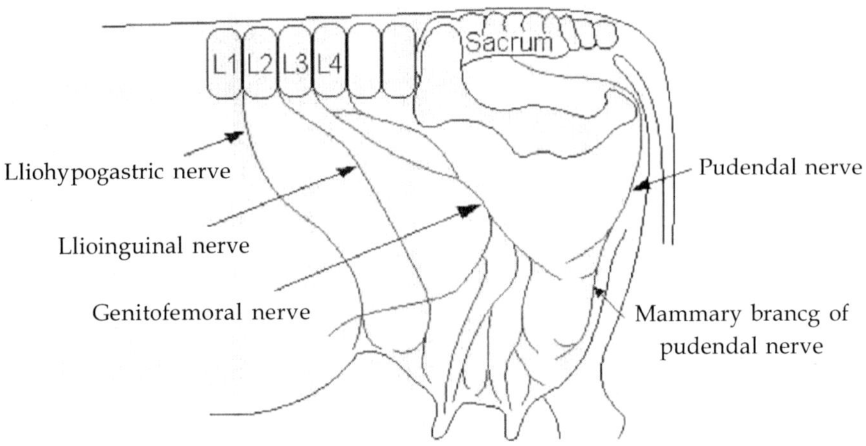

Figure. Nerve supply of the udder

The major innervations of udder has following nerves;

1. Ventral branch of 1st lumber nerve-Nerve from the first lumbar supply to the front part of udder but not the parenchyma.
2. Ventral branch of 2nd lumber Nerve- Second lumbar nerve also supply to the front/and lateral side of the udder.
3. Ventral component of inguinal Nerve
4. Dorsal component of inguinal Nerve
5. Inguinal Nerve
6. Antieror inguinal Nerve
7. Posterior inguinal Nerve
8. Perineal Nerve

The second nerve branch also anastomoses with the 3rd lumber nerve which then fences with the 4 and 5th lumber nerve and forms Inguinal Nerve. The inguinal nerve passes through the inguinal canal and innervates the parenchyma of udder and skin. It has both sensory and motor innervations. Inguinal nerves divide into anterior and posterior branches which supply to front and rear part of the udder. Sensory fibers send signals to the higher center which are sent back by efferent or motor fibre and non-ventral root ganglia to the mammary gland.

The role of nervous regulation in lactation or milk secretion is not very well understood as the transplanted mammary gland may also secrete milk. However, nervous system regulates the mammary secretion indirectly by altering the feed intake, water intake, release of hormones and stress mitigation. The act of milking also stimulate feed and water intake centre in hypthalamus suggesting a role of nervous system in lactation. The typical neuroendocrine reflex of let-down down of milk suggests the intricate relationship of nervous system with release of hormones. The poor feeding of cows leads to less milk yield and loss in body weight because of the regulation of feed and water intake by hypothalamus. Research experiments have proved that the lesions in ventromedial nucleus (VMN) induce hyperphagie or more feed intake while lesions in the lateral part of VMN lead to *anorexia,* indicating the role of hypothalamic "Appetite centers".

Another evidence of role of nervous regulation of milk secretion is release of galactopoitic hormones from the anterior pituitary glands which are essential either for milk synthesis (GH, PRL, Cortisol and Insulin) or milk removal (Oxytocin). Complete denervation of mammary glands in sheep and goat has no effect on milk ejection or milk production and no release of oxytocin. But in rabbit, denervation between mammary gland and brain leads to cessation of lactation and an injection of oxytocin, ACTH or PRL restores lactation. The milk synthesis in rats can occur in the absence of somatic sensory innervations, but intact spinal cord is essential. Intact somatic sensory innervations is necessary for milk secretion in cat. Spinal cord section leads to the cessation of milk secretion even if oxytocin is injected. Thus species variation exists for the necessity of spinal cord connections, between mammary gland and CNS. In sheep and goat innervation is not required where as rabbit needs only oxyocin for lactation. Rat has a limited secretion of oxytocin but it is missing in cats. The teat receives sensory nerve fibres which are concerned in the initiation of the milk-ejection reflex as well as sympathetic fibres which causes smooth muscles to contract.

The neurotransmitter released from parasympathetic nerves is known as acetylcholine while neuroendocrine components of sympathetic nerves release epinephrine and norepinephrine hormone. Epinephrine and nor-epinephrine are released primarily from medulla region of adrenal gland. Norepinephrine is also released as a neurotransmitter from peripheral nerves and nerves in the brain. The effect of sympathetic nerves on milk ejection depends upon the type of neurotransmitter receptor:

Generally,

- Alpha-receptors are vasoconstrictive in nature
- Nor-epinephrine can stimulate milk ejection via brain alpha-receptors
- Nor-epinephrine can inhibit milk ejection via brain beta-receptors
- Thus the location of these receptors determine the response
- There is no direct innervations of alveoli or myoepithelial cells.

There are no parasympathetic innervations in the mammary gland. However sensory receptors (neurons) are found in the teat. There are pressure-sensitive neurons around the gland and teat cisterns and the large milk collecting ducts. Hormone nor-epinephrine and epinephrine can inhibit oxytocin-induced contraction of myoepithelial cells which has been discussed in detail in oxytocin chapter. In the bovine species nor-epinephrine is the primary catecholamine. Injections of nor-epinephrine into cows increase blood flow to 2 to 5 times above normal and decrease milk yield.

❑❑❑

Chapter-7

Milk Secretion

Milk secretion is defined as the physiological process by which the milk constituents synthesized by the epithelial cells are released into the lumen of alveoli.

Source of milk constituents

Milk fat, protein and lactose component are synthesized by the epithelial cells of the alveoli but certain milk components like vitamins, minerals and few proteins are not synthesized in the mammary gland. These components are taken from the blood into the cells and then released into milk. Lactose, fat and most of the proteins are formed in the epithelial cells from the precursors supplied by the blood.

Secretion of milk constituents

The processes by which milk constituents (fat, protein etc.) are released from the epithelial cells into the lumen of the alveolus is called secretion. Milk fat is produced as small droplets within the epithelial cell. These droplets enlarge by merging together as they move towards apical part of the cell. The fat droplets are released from the epithelial cell by pinching off process. The fine apical membrane of the epithelial cell forms outer layer of the milk fat globule during milk secretion. Casein and lactose molecules are released in the form of secretory vesicles (SV) which are surrounded by a membrane. As in the case of fat, these vesicles move towards the apical part of cell and are released into lumen of the alveolus. Before being released the wall of SV fuses with cell membrane and the contents are then discharged into the alveolar cavity. This fusion of vesicle membrane and cell membrane repairs the loss caused by release of fat droplets. The secretion of fat and protein is a continous process and each epithelial cell may discharge fat or protein and casein 15 to 20 times between milkings.

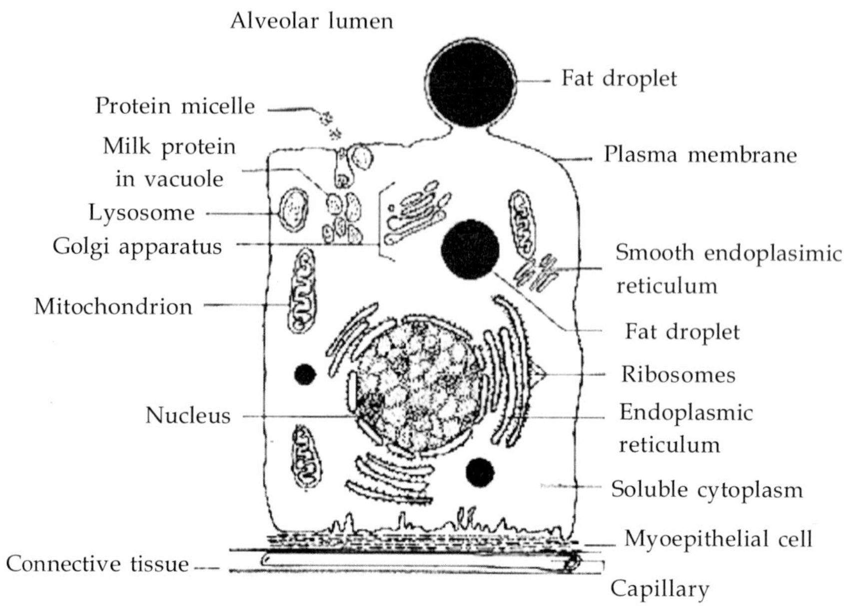

Figure. Release of fat and protein by an epithelial cell

The molecules of proteins, milk sugar, vitamins, and minerals are uniformally distributed within the milk. However, milk fat globules float in water after entering the lumen of alveolus. These fat droplets then collect as tiny clusters which cannot easily pass through the tiny ducts draining the alveoli. However, water moves freely along the ducts and gradually fills the cisterns of quarters. Some of the fat is even retained within the secretory cell and will escape only when pressure within the udder drops during milking. Thus milk removed from the udder initially contains only 1 to 2% fat, while subsequent milk may have more fat.

Milk secretion rate

The rate at which epithelial cells synthesize milk is high for the first 10 hours after milking. It starts declining afterwards. If a cow or buffalo is not milked, the milk synthesis and secretion will cease about 35 hours from the last milking. The milk secretory process stops due to increased pressure inside the alveolus. The high intramammary pressure constricts the blood vessels and stops the flow of blood and supply of milk precursors to the epithelial cells. Low producing cows are less adversely affected by long intervals between milkings as they have less secretory tissue in the udder. Consequently, the increase in udder pressure per unit milk is greater in younger and low producing cows. The short milking intervals are thus important for young cows. Incomplete milking by leaving 2 kg or more milk in the udder causes a permanent depression in the milk production.

Milk secretion is affected by many factors like parity, stage of lactation, milking interval, frequency of milking, residual milk and milking management practices. The rate of milk secretion is important in determining how much extra milk will be produced when cows are milked more often than twice daily. Milking of high producing cows (>12-15 kg/d) three times a day againt two times a day increases milk yield by 20%. Milking 4 times/day yields further 5 to 10% increase. However, when we take into consideration the feeding and labor cost, it is not economical and advisable. Three times milking is economical in case of cows producing more than 15 kg/d milk. Skipping one milking a week reduces the total milk yield by 5 to 10%. Milking of cows and buffaloes with medium production potential at regular milking interval of 12 hr. is an important practice in dairy farming under rural condtion. Agalactia is defined as a complete lactation failure while hypogalactia is partial failure of lactation.

Regulation of milk secretion by nervous system

The regulation of milk secretion by nervous system has not been elucidated extensively. Many studies indicate that frequent milking of dairy animals stimulates milk secretion.

Mammary glands respond to the following neural factors for milk synthesis.

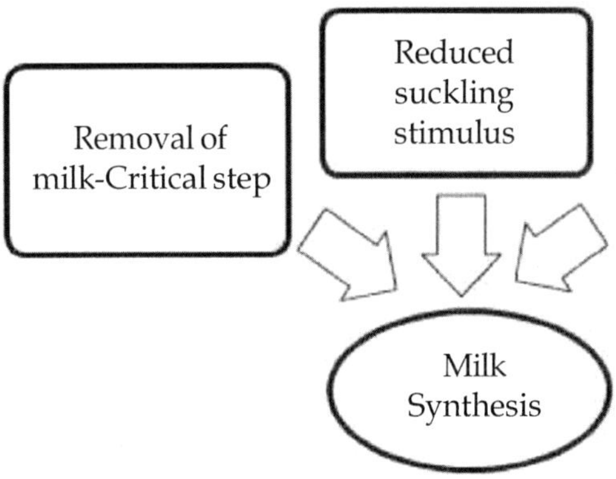

Effect of neural factors on milk synthesis

It has been reported that the nutritional demand of the pups or litter can modulate the production capacity of the mammary gland in rats. In ruminants, increased milking frequency (IMF) of ≥ 3 times or intense suckling by calf results in more synthesis of milk. Thus IMF can be used to augment milk production and production efficiency.

Frequent milking in dairy animals - The cows, milked 3 times in a day produce 15-20% more milk. Similarly 4 times milking is better than 3 times milking which leads to an additional increase of milk. This indicates that mammary gland is especially sensitive to the demand of offspring in early lactation which influence shape of lactation curve and persistency of lactation.

IMF in ruminants and rodents increases milk yield due to;

a) Increase in mammary cell number and

b) Mammary cell activity.

In addition to IMF the effect of suckling intensity on mammary gland development has also been reported.

In Rodents: Mammary development with more suckling is accompanied by an;

a) Increase in DNA

b) Increase in RNA

c) Increase in RNA:DNA ratio

Effect of IMF and suckling intensity on hormones

- Suckling causes release of prolactin and oxytocin in rodents. PRL stimulates mammary cell differentiation.
- Increasing the litter size leads to increase in PRL levels of pituitary gland.
- Increased PRL level is attributed to higher mammary cell activity.
- Injection of oxytocin in rat extends lactation due to complete evacuation of mammary gland but does not influence milk yield.
- Cortisol is the rate limiting factor during late lactation in rodents but injection of this hormone does not elicit a clear cut increase in the milk yield. It is suggested that local factors regulate the mammary response to the systemic hormones.

Local regulation of mammary functions

- Experiments carried out with selected teat ligation and suckling of intact teats by pups revealed that 24 hr milk stasis leads to reduction in RNA:DNA ratio by 31%, due to decreased mammary cell activity, increased intra-mammary pressure, engorgement of gland with milk and mammary gland involution. During suckling the mammary gland take up more nutrients which leads to the increased milk yield, mammary cell number and mammary cell activity. The local blood flow regulates all these events. When ligated glands are allowed to suckle by pups, the blood supply to the capillaries is restored, thus leading to the restoration of mammary function which suggests the role of blood flow rather than systemic hormones.
- In ruminants, the blood flow is inversely related to amount of milk accumulated in the gland. Milk stasis in cows decrease blood flow rate and decrease nutrient availability to the mammary glands. In goat, the mammary blood flow decreases linearly (51-70%) over 36 hr, due to negative feedback from the gland. However, IMF leads to increased blood flow in goats.

Effect on mammary development in ruminant

Milking frequency is positively related to milk production in cattle and therefore 3 times milking is practiced in the organized herd which is superior to 2 times milking. It has been found that beneficial effect of 3 times over the 2 times milking during the first few weeks of early lactation is carried over through the remainder of lactation. The 4 times milking over 2 times milking of cows during first 3 weeks of early lactation results in an increase of 8.8 kg/d milk and 2.6kg/d during the remainder lactation. Thus more milk can be obtained throughout lactation by putting an initial investment on labor for few weeks. The cellular responses to increased milking frequency for enhanced milk production are due to;

a) Increase in mammary cell number
b) Increase in mammary cell activity
c) Increase in activity of enzymes (protein and lactose)
d) Increase in alveolar area (increased cellular differentiation and proliferation)

However, increasing the milking frequency to 4 times during mid lactation (119-126 d) has no effect on the above attributes.

❑❑❑

Chapter-8

Mammogenesis

Mammary gland is an intriguing structure and its development (mammogenesis) is important from the production point of view. During the life time of an animal, mammary gland undergoes changes in size, structure, composition and secretory activity. The growth of mammary gland begins during fetal life and continues even after the mammary gland has reached its maturity. The mammary gland possesses secretory parenchyma cells together with supporting structure of connective and adipose tissue. Mammary glands have potential to produce milk more than its own weight every day or, in energetic terms, as many joules/day as it contains in its own mass. Mammogenesis begins in early stages of fetal life and continues after birth of calf during pre-puberty, puberty, pregnancy and lactation. Thus mammary gland undergoes growth, functional differentiation, and regression during initiation of lactation, pregnancy and the dry period. There are five distinct stages of mammary growth, namely;

a) Fetal development

b) Pre-pubertal development from birth to puberty

c) Post pubertal development during recurring estrous cycle

d) Growth during pregnancy and

e) Growth during lactation

The growth of mammary glands as a whole and of mammary epithelial cells in particular is influenced by hormones, nutrition and environment.

a. Fetal development of mammary gland

The development of mammary gland starts in early embryonic stage. The mammary gland is derived from the ectoderm and mesoderm. The cells of ectoderm get thickened on the ventral surface of embryo in the inguinal region between hind legs which results in the formation of mammary band at 30 days of age. Mammary band subsequently transform into mammary streak, line, crest and hillock at 34, 35, 37 and 40 days of embryonic age. Mammary hillock is a dome shape structure of ectodermal cells which grow into the mesenchymal layer. During further growth it gives rise to a spherical shape structure called mammary bud. The mammary bud is formed when embryo is about 2.1 cm long at 43 days of age. In the bovine species there are two mammary buds in the inguinal region on each side which gives rise to the fore and rear quarters.

Sex differentiation at the mammary bud stage

The development of mammary gland in males and females is similar upto the mammary bud formation. This stage marks the beginning of differentiation patterns and is the stage at which mammary gland of females and males can be distinguished by the following characteristics.

- Female mammary buds are ovoid while that of males are spherical in shape.
- Female mammary buds have a smaller volume than the males.
- Female mammary buds do not form as deep mammary pit as in males.
- Male's teat is pointed than the female which is flat on the end.
- There is no teat formation in male rats, mice, or horses. In other species, mammary development in male becomes slower than that of the female after the mammary bud stage.

The mammary bud is actually exteriorized, becomes separated from the epidermis and is eliminated in male mouse fetuses. As a result, no nipple or mammary structures are present in the newborn male mouse.

The development of teats begins by about 60 days when fetus is about 8 cm long in bovines. A rapid growth of mesenchyme tissue around the mammary bud raises the area containing the bud from the surrounding surface. Blood vessels begin to form in the mesenchyme during this stage. Invagination of the mammary bud cells into the mesenchyme push the mesenchymal cells aside and forms a solid core of cells called *primary sprout* by 80 days of embryonic age.

The primary sprout is a solid core of cells that gives rise to the gland cistern. The primary sprout makes teat pore during further developement. Each teat has one teat pore to drain out the milk in cows, buffaloes, sheep, goat, guinea pigs, rat, mice but 2 pore in horses, 3 pores in pigs, 6 pores in rabbit, 10 pores in dogs and 15 pores in humans. The mammry gland development is similar in male and female fetus upto primary sprout formation, but in males the surge of testosterone from fetal testis causes pinching off or pychosis of neck of primary sprout. This results in separation of it from mammary bud and leads to lack of teat formation in males. In such cases the primary sprout retained in mammary fat pad is viable to stimuls of estrogen and progesterone. The middle layer or mesoderm gives rise to connective tissue consisting of areolar tissue, fibrous tissue, elastic tissue and adipose tissue.

Secondary Sprouts –In bovine fetus, primary sprout gives rise to a number of the off-shoots or branches in the mesenchyme tissue which are called secondary sprouts at about 13-14 wks of age, just prior to the canalization of primary sprout. Secondary Sprouts are also solid core of epithelial cells which form the major ducts of mammary gland.

Canalization - The process of dissolution of cells and formation of a lumen in the solid core of epithelial cells in the primary and secondary sprouts is known as canalization. It begins at about 100 days of age in bovine fetus when it is about 19 cm long. As the circumference of the sprout increases the cells of central part does not receive adequate nourishment, dissolves and a lumen is formed. This begins at the proximal end of primary sprout and proceeds in both directions, forming the gland cistern. The secondary sprouts begin to open at the base and form the ducts of gland. Canalization proceeds back towards the surface and teat cistern are formed at about 130 days of age and finally the formation of streak canal takes place. Expansion and canalization continues until such canals are lined with only a couple of layers of epithelial cells.

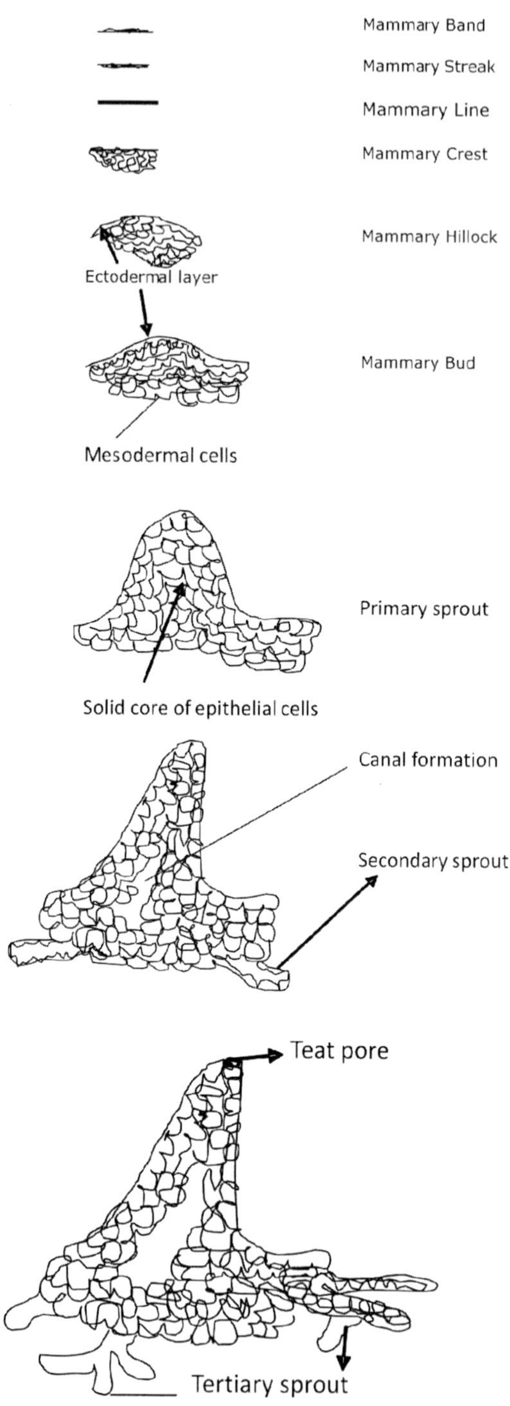

Figure. Stages of fetal development of mammary gland

a) Mammary gland development from birth to puberty

The mammary gland at birth has following characteristics.

- Basic structures of the mammary glands are formed in fetal life
- Rudimentary epithelial cells
- Few ducts cells adjacent to the gland cistern
- No alveoli
- Almost fully developed non-connective tissue (stromal and circulatory systems)
- Distinct outer shape of the mammary glands

After the birth of a neonate calf the following types of mammary growth occurs:

Isometric growth - After birth the growth of mammary gland continues and is referred as Isometric type of growth *i.e.* mammary gland grows at the same rate as general body growth. The non epithelial tissue grows for the first 2-3 months of isometric growth. During this phase following changes occur in the mammary gland;

a) Duct system enlarges a little.

b) Udder size increases due to increase in mammary fat pad and connective tissue.

c) Growth of mammary parenchyma is very little.

d) Growth of blood vessel takes place.

When the calf is about 75 days old, parenchyma tissue becomes evident at palpation and at 90 days of age, total parenchyma weighs about 10 g. However, at this stage no development of secretory alveoli occurs and the stroma cannot be separated from the parenchyma.

Allometric phase of growth- At about 2-3 months before the onset of puberty, the rate of mammary gland growth becomes 3.5 times faster than the rest of the body and is known as allometric phase of growth. This phase will not occur in absence of mammary fat pad and it lasts upto 12-14 months of age. During this phase following changes take place.

- Rapid growth of mammary fat pad till animals attains puberty
- Extensive growth and development of the duct network invades the surrounding adipose tissue (fat pad). The ducts need support

base of fat pad to grow. At this stage limitation of mammary fat pad will limit the growth of ducts. Formation of a duct network continues until heifers attain puberty. The mammary fat pad and the ductal network determine the extent of lobulo-alveolar growth during gestation.

- Alveoli are not formed.
- Mammary mass mainly contains fat pad during prepubertal period.

The allometric phase of growth in heifers is closely linked to the gradual maturation of ovaries. Mammary gland again returns to isometric type of growth coinciding with onset of puberty or shortly thereafter. At the end of allometric growth, the mammary gland of heifers weighs about 2-3 kg and contain about 0.5-1.0 kg parenchyma.

Attributes	Heifer	Lactating cow
Weight of mammary gland, kg	2.5-3.0kg	25.0 kg
Connective tissue, %	40-50	40
Epithelium, %	10-20	40-50
Fat, %	30-40	—
Lumen, %	—	15-20

The onset of puberty in exotic dairy heifers is achieved between 9 to 11 months of age at body weight of 250 to 280 kg. However, Indigeneous cattle heifers exhibit onset of puberty between 17-20 months. In many studies, attempts have been made to predict the future milk yield from birth to 6 months of age by palpation of gland in mature animals but this method is not reliable. The methods to measure mammary gland growth includes following parameters.

- Tissue weight
- Tissue area
- DNA content (indicative of epithelial cell numbers)
- Incorporation of [^{3}H] thymidine into DNA (indicative of cell division)
- RNA content (indicative of protein synthetic capacity)
- Hydroxyproline (as a way of measuring connective tissue content) and
- Total lipid content

Milk production potential of heifers or a lactating cow could be related to these parameters. In heifers, the correlation between mammary DNA or RNA and subsequent milk production is low (0.25). In rats, the correlation between mammary DNA and RNA at puberty and subsequent litter weight gains are 0.34 and 0.57, respectively.

b. Post-pubertal development (Recurring estous cycle)

The growth of the mammary gland after attainment of puberty is controlled by sex steroid hormones released from the ovary and the hormones from anterior pituitary gland. Progesterone and estrogen stimulate ductal and lobule-alveolar growth in mammary gland. The growth of ducts, their branching and lengthening takes place with a combination of estrogen, prolactin and GH. The ductal elongation and branching invade the mammary fat pad by actively growing structures called *Terminal End Buds* (TEB). These end buds represent the structures where elongation and branching of the ducts takes place by estrogen stimulated cell division. Estrogen causes cell multiplication at the tip of the TEB and enlargement of ducts (lengthening and branching of ducts), while progesterone causes duct and ductule cells to multiply, leading to ductule development and duct widening. TEBs are not present in ruminants where fundamental developmental unit in the mamamry tissue is terminal ductule lobular unit (TDLU). A TDLU is a developmental and functional unit in the parenchymal tissue. Epithelial components of a TDLU are held together by loose intralobular connective tissue and are surrounded by a dense interlobular connective tissue sheath. TDLU grows to form a cluster of alveoli or lobuloalveolar unit during pregnancy. Mammary stromal cells in the region of the TEB or TDLU may be involved in dissolving the collagen so that mammary structures can expand. The enlarging ducts may promote mesenchyme growth and development of blood vessels called angiogenesis.

The receptors of estrogen and progesterone develop around puberty when mammary gland is exposed to cyclic elevations in estrogen and progesterone blood concentrations. Cyclic changes of these hormones during estrous cycles results mainly in duct elongation and some lobular tissue formation, but formation of alveoli does not occur. Effects of many mammogenic hormones are mediated through stroma-derived growth factors which act in a paracrine manner by eliciting mitogenic responses in the adjacent epithelial structures. In rodents, estrogen acts on its receptors in the stromal tissue and stimulate production of growth factors which in turn stimulate ductal development. The studies in cattle also indicate that estrogen action on mammary development may be mediated through the stroma.

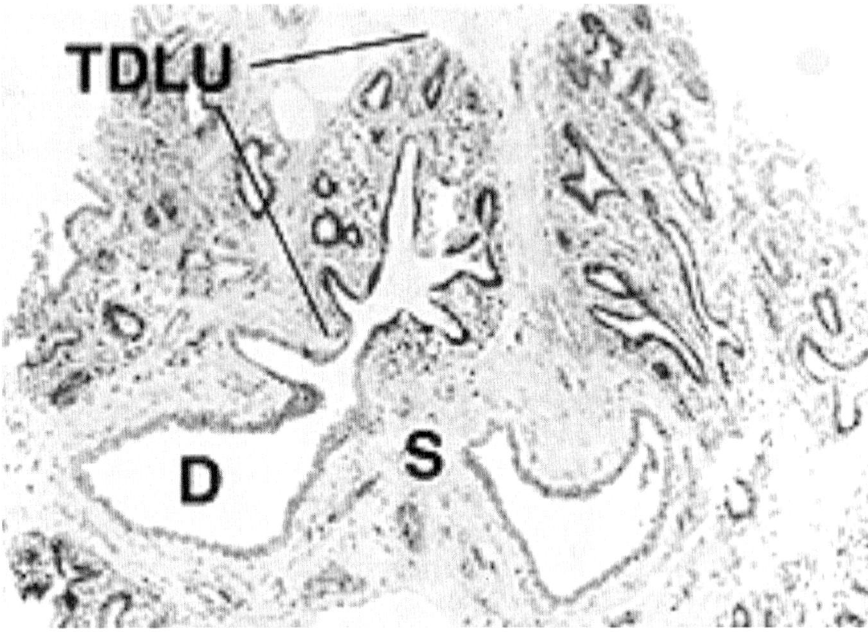

Progesterone plays a key role in mammary development though its receptors have been difficult to identify in the mammary fat pad. Administration of progesterone can results in proliferation of stromal cells under some physiological conditions. The effect of progesterone is mediated through binding to its receptors in epithelial cells and stimulating ductal side-branching or alveolar bud formation, which are the hallmarks of postpubertal mammary development. Estrogen also stimulates progesterone receptor expression in epithelial cells. Progesterone, therefore, has a major role in alveolar morphogenesis and a lesser role in ductal morphogenesis. During estrous cycles, duct elongation and expansion of the parenchymal tissue into the mammary fat pad occurs in limited bursts coinciding to elevated estrogen level. During luteal phase of elevated progesterone, relatively little further expansion occurs. Due to asynchronomous level of estrogen and progesterone hormone the growth of mammary gland is negligible during recurring estrous cycle. The developed alveoli is not in a good shape and may have irregular shape with folded epithelial layer.

c. Growth during pregnancy

The growth of mammary gland during pregnancy is extensive and is controlled by hormones released from ovary, pituitary and adrenal gland. During early pregnancy, the growth of mammary gland is less but it accelerates with advancement of pregnancy. Progesterone level remain elevated throughout gestation, while estrogen is elevated only during the later phase of gestation which coincides with greatest increases in mammary tissue mass. Synergy between estrogen and progesterone is observed during pregnancy and elevated blood concentrations of estrogen and progesterone together establish the conditions required for the exponential mammary cell growth. The extensive lobulo-alveolar development and growth of ducts increases mammary gland mass during pregnancy. The adipose tissue of the mammary fat pad is replaced by the blood vessels, ducts, connective tissue and the growing alveoli. Thus alveoli are formed only when pregnancy is established in cows and buffaloes. The effects of estrogen and progesterone on the mammary glands are also mediated by autocrine and paracrine factors which are produced locally in the mammary tissue. Estrogen may have indirect effect through their impact on prolactin secretion. The mammary gland remodels extensively during pregnancy leading to more rapid extension and branching of the ductal structure. The alveolar development brings out an increase in tissue nutrition requirement and is accompanied by substantialvascular remodeling. Growth of new blood vessels occur during this stage of mammary development. Vascular growth is a requirement for alveolar development and milk production. The growth of new blood vessels and formation of vascular tissue is regulated by growth factors like;

- Vascular endothelial growth factor (VEGF)
- Angiopoietin and
- Ephrin families

The role of VEGF in angiogenesis during alveolar differentiation is still unclear. VEGF is up-regulated by prolact in the principal hormone driving mammary development in advance of lactation. VEGF-A, the principal member of the VEGF family is a multifunctional cytokine that stimulates angiogenesis, increases vascular permeability to water and proteins, causes vasodilatation and formation of fenestrations in endothelial cells. Recent experiments on mice with a conditional VEGF gene inactivation in alveolar-myoepithelial cells have demonstrated that milk production is dependent on VEGF production by myoepithelial cells.

d. Growth during lactation

Growth of the mammary gland continues to occur after the parturition during early lactation. The continuous increasing milk yield trend till attainment of peak yield in 2-8 weeks indicates more metabolic activity and increased number of epithelial cells. The rapid growth of mammary gland during last few days of pregnancy that does not stop abruptly following parturition, however after peak lactation the number of secretory cells begin to decline. Thus peak milk yield is dependent on the number of milk secreting epithelial cells. Persistency of lactation or maintaining the peak milk yield depends on the continual survival of milk secreting epithelial cells. Intensive research on mammary growth during lactation is required to explicit the role of hormones and non-hormonal factors in mammogenesis. In rats, proliferation of cells during early lactation may account for as much as three-quarters of the increase in daily milk yield between parturition and peak lactation; the remainder is due to the increased activity of existing cells. Conversely, in goats, the entire initial decline in milk yield after peak lactation is attributed to the loss of secretory cells. Increased frequency of milking enhances milk yield and reduces secretory cell loss in cows and buffaloes.

Endocrine regulation of mammogenesis

There are 2 categories of hormones involved in the regulation of mammary gland development.

1. Reproductive hormones like estrogen, progesterone, placental lactogen, prolactin and oxytocin that directly influence mammary gland growth.
2. Metabolic hormones- The important hormones in this regard are growth hormone, corticosteroids, thyroid hormone, insulin, and leptin. These hormones regulate metabolic responses to nutrient intake or stress; often have direct effects on the mammary gland.

1. Prolactin (PRL)

Prolactin, produced from the anterior pituitary gland, is a single-chain polypeptide hormone with a molecularweight of 23 kD. Extra pituitary PRL is produced in the brain, lung, adrenals, islets of Langerhans, skin, prostate, testis, ovary, decidua, and immune system including lymphocytes and mammary gland. The best known action of PRL on the mammary gland is,

- Initiation of lactation or lactogenesis and maintenance of lactation or galactopoiesis
- Regulation of mammary gland development and differentiation or mammogenesis

The receptors of prolactin are present in the mammary fat pad in some species and in mammary epithelium.Due to this reason, prolactin may act on both epithelial and stromal components of the growing mammary tissue. Inhibition of prolactin secretion inhibits mammary gland development in pregnant goats, pigs and other species. Blood concentrations of prolactin are normally maintained at low level during pregnancy. Thus mammary development during pregnancy may not be limited by the normal blood concentrations of prolactin. Mammary epithelial cells of pregnant and lactating rat synthesize local PRL. But significance of local extra-pituitary PRL production, its regulation and functions have not been determined in detail as yet. PRL mRNA in the rat mammarygland is expressed during pregnancy and lactation. PRL mRNA expressionis initiated in mid to late pregnancy in parallel with the development of mammary gland and declines in the early phase of weaning with the regression of the mammary gland. The mammary gland growth is also affected by photoperiod.

Mammary growth is stimulated by 16: 8hr. light: dark cycle as compared to 8: 16, in prepubertal and postpubertal heifers. The replacement and ablation experiments using ergot drugs provide evidence that increased periparturient secretion of prolactin is necessary for maximal milk production in cattle. Quantitative microscopy indicates that a relative mammary epithelial cells differentiation fails in cows inhibited for secretion of prolactin. Prolactin induces synthesis and secretion of alpha-lactalbumin in prepartum bovine mammary tissue. Temporary disruption of mammary microtubules immediately pre-partum in pregnant heifers reduces subsequent milk production, biosynthetic capacity and cellular differentiation. For maximal milk production, mammary secretory cells apparently must respond to lactogenic hormone stimulation during the immediate periparturient period.

2. Growth hormone

Growth hormone influence mammary growth even in fetal stages. Growth hormone or somatotropin administration stimulates milk production during lactation in cattle and buffaloes. Daily injection of somatotropin from 8 to 15.6 months of age in heifers increases mammary parenchyma and decreases extra-parenchymal tissue. Growth hormone can stimulate mammary growth at all stages of development through increased hepatic synthesis of insulin-like growth factor i.e. IGF-1, which is a potent mitogen for mammary cells. Therefore, growth hormone may be a major factor in the control of mammary development during the prepartum period. Growth hormone administration during the prepubertal period does not increase milk yield in first lactation. Prepartum administration of rBST slow release formulation (160 mg/14d) enhances milk production in the following lactation due to more mammary gland development. Mammary parenchyma is positively correlated with GH levels. There is evidence for growth hormone receptors in mammary epithelial or stromal cells in various species. Growth hormone may act on ruminant mammary tissue by stimulating stromal production of IGF-I which is mitogenic for mammary epithelial cells. It has been found that the highest level of IGF-I expression occurs in the mammary fat pad during the prepubertal allometric growth phase and during late pregnancy. Mammary expression of IGF-I is regulated by growth hormone, estrogen and positive feedback stimulation from proliferating epithelial cells. The role of IGF-II in mammary growth is less clear than that of IGF-I. Stromal cells probably produce IGF-II which is regulated by stages of mammary development. Recent studies suggests that GH and IGF-I mediate glandular development together with estrogen.

3. Leptin

Another protein hormone is leptin that influences mammary gland development due to excessive fattening. This hormone is produced and secreted predominantly by white adipose tissue or WAT. It has a critical role in the regulation and coordination of energy metabolism. Identification of leptin in the milk of several mammals and humans indicate regulatory effect of this hormone in cow mammary gland. The expression of leptin receptor in culture of lactating mammary tissue increases approximately 25 times by prolactin, but had no effect on virgin calf mammary tissue. Leptin-enhances fatty acid synthesis in the presence of prolactin, but had no effect without presence of prolactin. Leptin decreases IGF-1-induced bovine mammary cell proliferation and inhibits IGF-1 signaling through stimulation of macrophages. Macrophages increase their phagocytic activity and production of cytokines like TNF and IL-6 which inhibits IGF-1-induced proliferation in other cell types.

4. Placental lactogen

Placental lactogens (PL) are synthesized and secreted from the placenta of many species. PL has prolactin and growth hormone-like activity depending upon the species. In pregnant goats, the concentration of placental lactogen in the maternal blood is closely correlated with the number of fetus. This graded concentration of placental lactogen, in combination with other mammogenic hormones, may regulate the extent of mammary development during late pregnancy. In dairy cows, a relationship between placental mass and subsequent milk production has been found. However, concentration of placental lactogen in maternal blood of the dairy cow is low and the effect of placental mass may result from other placental hormones including estrogen. Pigs and rabbits do not have a placental lactogen. Increased level of PL in late pregnancy relates to mammary growth, calf size and milk production and the effects are mediated by local IGF-I. However, PL may have little direct effect on mammary growth or lactogenesis.

5. Adrenal steroid

Glucocorticoids are also required for the mammary growth during pregnancy especially during late lactation. The effect of glucocorticoids is direct and indirect. The indirect effects are due to their involvement in nutrient metabolism. In early gestation corticoid binding globulin (CBG) concentration is more that binds with the glucocorticoids and thus free hormone is not available to act on mammary gland. But during late lactation, cortisol concentration increases mainly due to less CBG and contribution of fetal cortisol. The cortisol hormone is required for both ductal growth and lobulo-alveolar differentiation. However, these changes around parturition are associated with the lactogenesis.

6. Other hormones

Hormones like thyroid hormones, insulin and relaxin are also required for mammary cell growth. Insulin synergizes with estrogen and progesterone to increase mammary development but normal blood concentrations of insulin are not rate limiting for normal mammary development. Relaxin hormone is associated with the parturition process, uterine cervix dilation or nipple development during rat pregnancy. It has a minor role in growth and differentiation of rat mammary gland. However, it plays a major role in sow, while its role in mammogenesis in cows and buffaloes remains to be elucidated.

7. Autocrine and paracrine factors

Autocrine and paracrine factors or local growth factors play a major role in mammary growth. Many effects of steroid hormones on mammary growth are mediated by local growth factors like TGFα, TGF-β, EGF, FGF, HGF and KGF at the mammary tissue level. These include an interaction between the developing mammary epithelial structures and the mammary fat pad. Mammary epithelial cells will only grow and organize when transplanted into the fat pad. The interaction may involve specific fatty acids from the fat pad which may induce changes in epithelial development. Local production of transforming growth factor-β (TGF-β) inhibits mammary growth such as during the pre-pubertal period and between estrous cycles. Epidermal growth factor (EGF) and transforming growth factor-alpha (TGF-α) produced in the mammary tissue stimulate mammary cell proliferation. EGF and TGF-α both bind to the EGF receptors. The mammogenic action of estrogen and progesterone hormone occurs in part by decreasing local production of TGF-β and increased local production of TGF-α and increasing EGF receptor in mammary epithelium. Stromal EGF receptors are also necessary for normal ductal growth. Growth factors like hepatocyte growth factor (HGF), fibroblast growth factor (FGF) family such as acid-FGF and Keratinocyte growth factor (KGF) are known epithelial cell mitogens being produced by stromal cells. These may be involved in mediating the effects of mammogenic hormones. Basic-FGF also is an epithelial cell mitogen, but origin of this growth factor in the mammary tissue is uncertain.

Importance of mammary fat pad

Mammary fatty pad arises from the mesoderm during the embryonic development and is essential for the growth of mammary gland in species such as cattle, goat and sheep in which mammary gland is in close proximity to the scrotum of the male fetus. In such cases fatty pad has no room to proliferate which leads to the termination of mammogenesis at early stages of development. The mammary fat pad provide the basic network support for development of mammary epithelium, provides signals that mediate ductal morphogenesis and probably alveolar differentiation. It is also established that stromal tissue and epithelial element interact for mammary glandular development through cytokines. Stromal cells appear to influence the epithelial cell behavior by secretion of growth factors and by altering the composition of extracellular matrix protein (fibronectin, collagen and lamina). Extracellular matrix components which are important for mammary tissue growth and function are produced by both epithelial cells and stromal cells.

Recent studies suggest that GH and IGF-I mediate glandular development together with estrogen. Experiment carried out in the female hyphophysectomised and oophorectomized rat with bGH alone or with Estrogen *i.p.* indicate that GH stimulate IGF-I mRNA concentration in gland free mammary fat pad. GH acts synergistically with estradiol in induction of IGF-I mRNA. Mammary epithelial structures often grow into a lipid-rich environment of the fat pad. Fatty acids, particularly unsaturated fatty acids, stimulate mammary epithelial cell growth and can substantially enhance the in-vitro effects of other growth factors such as IGF-I and EGF. Mammary stromal cells are also involved in dissolving the connective tissue collagen, so that epithelial structures can continue to grow. Several proteases involved in tissue remodeling and growth of parenchymal tissue are derived from stromal tissue.

Role of nutrition in mammary gland development

Milk production is a function of number of secretory cells present in the mammary gland. Therefore, factors that determine the size of epithelial cell population have an impact on milk production. Mammary growth can be affected by nutrition, hormones, growth factors, and cytokines. The most important nutrient factor is the daily energy intake or feeding level. Feeding levels with daily body weight gains of >700 g/day in heifers adversely influence the growth of mammary parenchyma. Many authors have implicated possible role of GH in high energy level fed heifers. High feeding level reduces GH levels which lowers the growth of mammary gland. Mammary gland growth seems to be sensitive to negative effect of high feeding level at 3 months of age; however, it is not possible to separate out the effect of energy and protein on mammary gland development. Thus the effect of high plane of nutrition is limited to pre-pubertal growth period only and does not influence post-pubertal growth. Nutrition can stimulate greater rates of lean gain during 2-3 months of age of calf without impairing future mammary development. Greater energy and protein intake to promote average daily gain of 0.66 kg/d during this period increases mammary parenchyma mass, DNA and RNA and epithelial cell proliferation. Increase in energy and protein intake results in greater mammary gland development between 2-8 week-old Holstein heifer calves, but does not stimulate additional growth of mammary parenchyma tissue in 8-to-14 wk-old calves. Excessive feeding only stimulates extra-parenchymal fat deposition. Mammary parenchyma tissue is positively correlated with GH levels and negatively correlated with mammary adipose tissue. The mammary growth is affected by specific components of the diet alone. Addition of poly-unsaturated fat in the diet increases mammary growth due to more growth hormone and prolactin receptors in liver and increased IGF-I level in blood.

❑❑❑

Chapter-9

Lactogenesis

Lactogenesis involves the cellular and biochemical changes whereby mammary epithelial cells are converted from a non-secretory to a secretory state. In other terms mammary epithelial cells acquire the ability to synthesize and secrete milk constituents. Lactogenesis involves two distinct stages.

Stage I: This stage involves following cytological and enzymatic differentiation in the alveolar epithelial cells.

- Increased synthesis of the enzymes like acetyl CoA carboxylase, fatty acid synthetase and the enzymes associated with the synthesis of other milk constituents
- Increased uptake and transport of precursors like amino acids, glucose for milk synthesis
- The synthesis of α-lactalbumin and lactose does not begin until stage II of lactogenesis approches. Thus formation of colostrum and uptake of immunoglobulins increases in mammary gland during this stage.

Stage II: The copious secretion of all milk constituents take place during this stage. In cows and buffaloes secretion is more from day -4 to few days postpartum. This phase is initiated by abolition of inhibitory effects of progesterone on lactogenesis i.e. about 2 days prepartum. The secretion of milk is further stimulated by very high blood prolactin and glucocorticoids levels around parturition. Thus a combination of lactogenic hormones i.e. increased glucocorticoids+ prolactin and decreased progesterone levels lead to transcription of the α-lactalbumin gene. The α-lactalbumin mRNA is translated at the rough endoplasmic reticulum (RER) and the α-lactalbumin enzyme interacts with galactosyl-transferase enzyme in the Golgi apparatus to synthesize lactose. Synthesis lactose osmotically draws water into the Golgi and secretory vesicles. This process allows the secretion of large amount of milk and is the most obvious manifestation of stage II of lactogenesis. At the same time, synthesis of other milk constiutents also increases.

Blood progesterone concentrations do not decline until parturition in women. Due to this reason the full impact of stage II lactogenesis sometimes does not occur until about 2 days postpartum. In pigs and mice, stage II of lactogenesis is occurring immediately prior to and at the time of parturition. In sow it is difficult to get any mammary secretion until parturition but in cows and buffaloes substantial mammary secretion can be obtained upto several days prepartum.

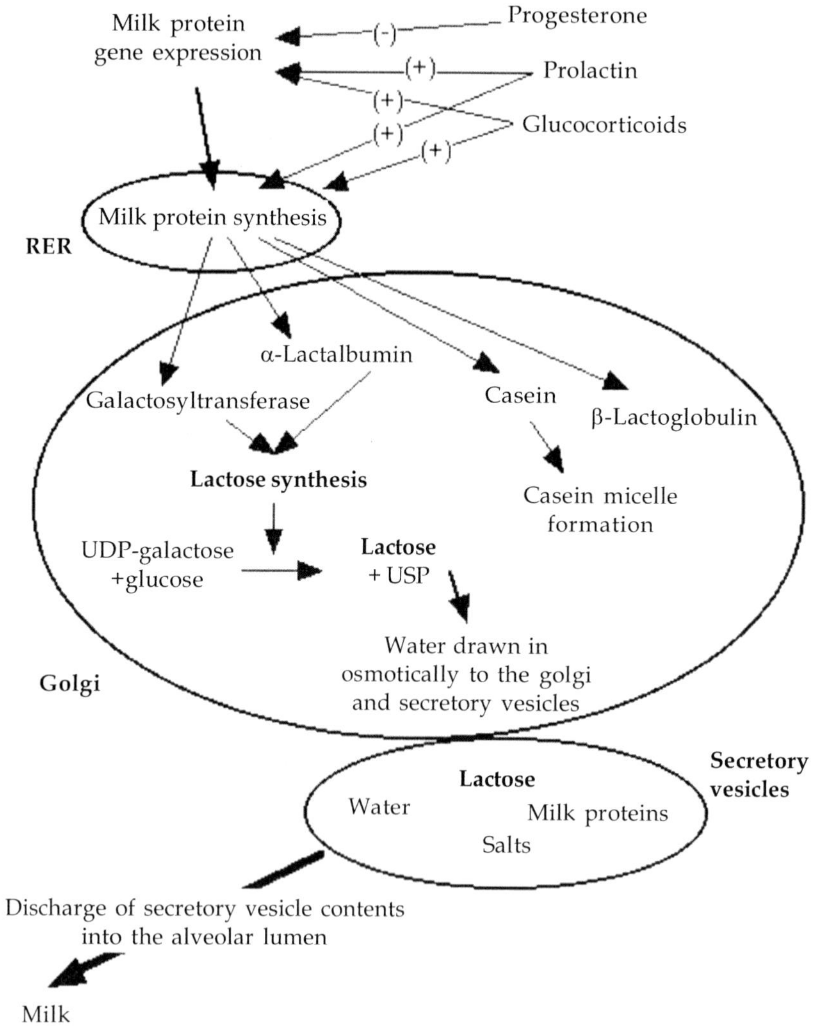

Figure. Role of hormones in lactogenesis

The mammary gland has a capacity to synthesize milk during late pregnancy stage, but the copious milk secretion takes place only near parturition. The mammary gland seems to be locked into a state where milk secreting cells are present during late pregnancy, but copious milk secretion cannot take place. Low levels of caseins and β-lactoglobulin are synthesized in the mammary cells during last trimester of pregnancy. Milk fat accumulates in the cells and alveoli during the final few days of pregnancy. But little synthesis of α-lactalbumin occurs until the immediate peripartum period.

Hormonal regulation of lactogenesis

Several hormones are involved in the initiation of lactation but hormones released from the pituitary gland, ovary and adrenal glands play an important role. Hormones of the anterior pituitary like GH and prolactin are involved in lactogenesis and their role in conjuction with other hormones have been established in various species. Hypophysectomy of pregnant animals suppresses lactation without affecting delivery of calf. The administration of crude pituitary extract initiates and maintains lactation in different species.

- Hypophysectomy in goats reduces milk yield.
- Injection of Glucocorticoids + T_3 + GH restore lactation (25%).
- Injection of prolactin in the above treatment restores lactation fully.

Prolactin: Prolactin plays a crucial role in initiation of lactation in cows, buffaloes and goats. The effect of prolactin on lactogenesis is highly species specific. For example, rabbit mammary gland is highly sensitive to prolactin hormone than any other species. Administration of prolactin or aqueous extract of pituitary produces more milk in Rabbit. However, prolactin does not initiate milk secretion due to luteotrophic property in rat and mice because of increased progesterone levels. Administration of bromocryptine, an ergot alkaloid abolishes the peak of prolactin at parturition and also results in low postpartum milk yield in cows, buffaloes and goats. The decreased yield is due to the decrease in metabolic activity of epithelial cells and not the cell numbers. Treatment with bromocryptine+ exogenous prolactin does not result in reduction of milk yield and confirms the role of prolactin in copious secretion of milk during stage-II of lactogenesis.

Prolactin hormone can regulate its own receptor numbers. The increase in prolactin concentration increases the number of PRLreceptors on the epithelial cells and the process is known as Up-regulation. The prolactin concentration remains low during pregnancy and increases before parturition coinciding to stage II of lactogenesis in small and large ruminants. The up-regulation of PRL is associated with the cell organelles differentiation. However sharp increases in prolactin, decreases its own receptors on the plasma membrane of epithelial cells and the process is called down-regulation.

Growth Hormone

The role of GH has been established in mammogenesis in many species including cows and buffaloes. The increase in GH levels before parturition has been correlated with mammary growth rather than with the milk secretion. Administration of rBST @160mg/14 d stimulate mammogenesis and postpartum yields in buffaloes. Abolition of peak of prolactin by bromocryptine results in compensatory release of GH on the day of parturition, but postpartum yields still remain low in buffaloes. Thus GH appears to act synergistically with prolactin.

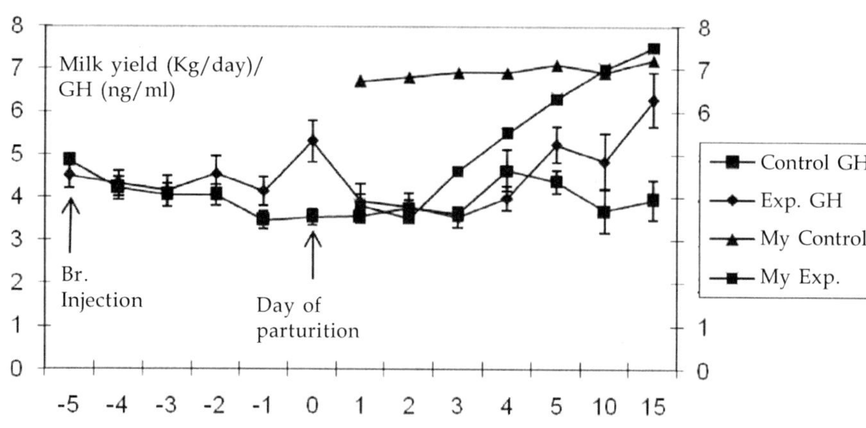

Figure. Effect of bromocryptine on plasma GH and milk yield in buffaloes

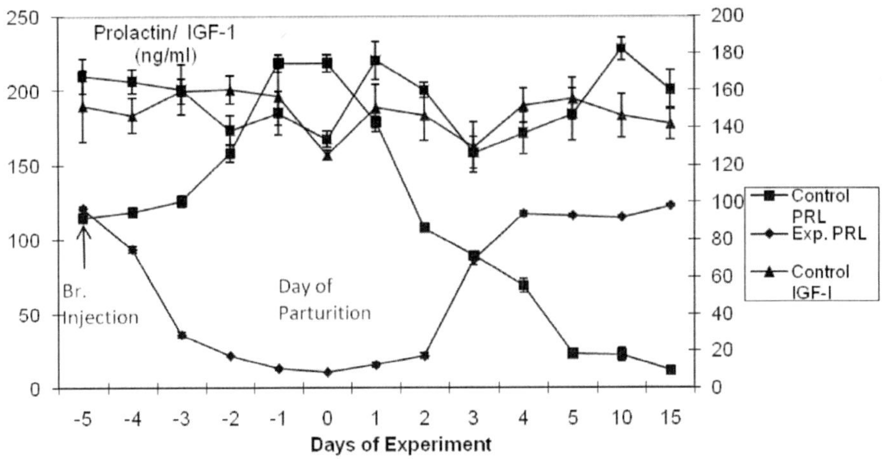

Fig. Plasma prolactin and IGF-I changes in buffaloes administered bromocryptine before parturition

Adrenal gland

The hormones of adrenal gland *i.e.*glucocorticoids play a major role in lactogenesis. Cortisol induces synthesis of casein like protein and mRNA, differentiation of Golgi apparatus and endoplasmic reticulum. Plasma cortisol level remains low during most part of the pregnancy, begin to increase-7 days prepartum and acquire peak level on day of parturition. The prepartum rise in cortisol levels are due to the less number of cortisol binding globulins (CBG) and contribution of fetal cortisol to maternal plasma. The following experiments also confirm the role of cortisol in lactogenesis.

a) Adrenalectomy of pregnant cows inhibits lactogenesis and subsequent lactation.

b) A combination of ACTH (glucocorticoids) + PRL initiates lactation in adrenalectomized and hypophysectomized animals.

c) Administration of glucocorticoids in pregnant cows initiates milk secretion.

Progesterone

Progesterone is one of the most important hormone associated with lactogenesis. Progestrone levels are higher during pregnancy and inhibit the onset of lactogenesis. This hormone is released from the corpus luteum to maintain the pregnancy and the lactation cannot be initiated unless its concentrations decrease to the minimum. Progesterone is also secreted by placenta during pregnancy. Progesterone concentration decline on day -2 to -1 and coincide with the stage II of lactogenesis. Injection of progesterone during pregnancy inhibits lactogenesis. Thus during preganancy initiation of milk secretion is checked by;

- Prevention of lactose synthesis
- Prevention of α-lactalbumin and casein synthesis
- Blocking of prolactin induced increase in milk constituents and accumulation of casein mRNA.
- Reduction in the ability of prolactin to induce synthesis of α-lactalbumin
- Disturb the synergism between prolactin and estrogen
- Competing with the receptors of glucocorticoids in cytoplasm and saturating its binding sites.
- Inhibiting the ability of prolactin to induce its own receptor called up-regulation.

Estrogen

The concentration of estrogen remains constantly low during most part of pregnancy and begins to increase one month prior to parturition. The highest level of estrogen reaches on day-2 of parturition and decline postpartum. Thus the change in estrogen signifies its role during both the phases of lactogenesis. Administration of estrogen in animals with well developed mammary gland induces milk secretion in many species by stimulating secretion of prolactin. In-vitro studies of mammary glands have shown that estrogen also stimulate synthesis of casein and α-lactalbumin.

Placental lactogen

During pregnancy, placenta secretes placental lactogen (PL) which have GH and PRL like activity. The increased concentration of PL coincides with the first phases of lactogeneis. PL may be involved in cellular differentiation of mammary glands as it also contributes in the initiation of lactation in many species. Rabbit and Pig placenta does not secrete PL, but its administration in rabbit stimulates milk secretion. In cows the placental cotyledons are lactogenic.

Prostaglandins

Prostglandins are produced locally in the tissues and these are derivatives of archidonic acid. Of all the prostaglandins, PGF-2α is the most potent luteolytic agent. Due to this reason administration of PGF2α during pregnancy lyses the corpus luteum and milk secretion begins. PGF2α concentration remains low during pregnancy but prepartum increased level of PGF2α coincides with decline in progesterone levels. The increased estrogen levels before parturition stimulate PGF2α release but precise role of PGF2α in lactogenesis has not been established.

Insulin

The insulin hormone has been shown to correlate with the milk protein synthesis. This hormone dramatically decline at the onset of lactation and remain low till 60 day post-partum when animal attain peak milk yield. This phase of insulinemia follows the pattern of milk protein concentration during lactation. The role of insulin in protein synthesis has been demonstrated in mice and cows.

Leptin

Leptin is synthesized in the adipose tissue. This hormone is considered as a potential candidate biomarker of milk yield, fat and protein content in cows. Leptin is secreted in the mammary glands during lactation and is also found in the colostrum of livestock species. Although it is primarily associated with appetite regulation, leptin and its receptors are expressed in the mammary gland so it may also act locally to influence mammary development It is considered that leptin level inform CNS about energy reserves and demand of animal to ensure successful lactation.

❑❑❑

Chapter-10

Induced Lactation

A number of elite cows and buffaloes suffer from repeat breeding problem due to abnormal parturition, metritis and dystocia. The animals which are inseminated atleast 4-5 times and do not conceive are declared as repeat breeders. High producing and elite animals usually suffer from such problems. As a result of culling these animals, a very high potential germ plasm is lost. Farmers also dispose of such cows and buffaloes due to high cost of rearing without getting any productive output or milk. The knowledge and role of estrogen and progesterone in mammary glands development has led to the application of both the hormones in artificial development of mammary glands. The artificial induction of lactation has been successfully achieved in exotic cows by the administration of estrogen and progestoerne in the ratio of 1:2.5, @ 0.1 mg per kg body wt. per day for a period of 7 days. Following a gap of another 7 days (8-14 d) the udder and teat message is done for 2-5 min. in the morning and evening hours for 7 days followed by milking on day 22 of the initiation of treatment. The udder and teat message of the cows release lactogenic hormones like prolactin, cortisol and GH which stimulates mammogenesis in conjunction with estrogen and progesterone hormone. The teats and udder are engorged with lacteal secretion on day 20 and 21. If udder engorgement is not fully achieved the massage could continue for 2- 3 days more and the cows may be milked on day 24-25. The crossbred cows can produce a very good quantity of milk with a success rate of 70-75 % by using this protocol. Researchers have advocated the use of reserpine, but photoperiodic duration is not a limitation under Indian conditions. Therefore, the use of reserpine should be avoided. The adverse effects of reserpine have also been reported in induced lactation. Indigenous cows and buffaloes give less milk yield with the same protocol. Administration of estrogen and progesterone in the ratio of 1:1 @0.1 mg/kg body wt./d for a period of 7 days have been found to induce mammary gland development and induction of lactation in indigenous Tharparkar cow and buffaloes (Table). The induced animals are teat messaged from 14 to 21 days and the milking can be done on day 24 of treatment. The hormones like GH, T4 and T3 are utilized by the developing mammry gland. Such cows and buffaloes secrete about 60-80 % of the total yield of previous lactation. The induced animals exhibit heat symptoms and the conception rate is 50 %. The milk composition in the treated animals becomes normal within a week. The pattern of change in the milk yield (lactation curve) of the induced primiparous and multiparous buffalo has been depicted in the figure.

Table. Mean plasma hormone changes in a Tharparkar cow induced into lactation with estrogen and progesterone hormone in the ratio of 1:1 for a period of 7 days.

Attributes	Periods of sampling			CD at 5%
	Before treatment	After steroid treatment	After start of milking	
Insulin (uU/ml)	23.12	27.70	24.21	–
GH (ng.ml)	4.49	2.08	1.09	1.26
T_4(ng/ml)	102.70	54.49	45.34	20.12
T_3(ng/ml)	2.66	1.59	1.54	0.49

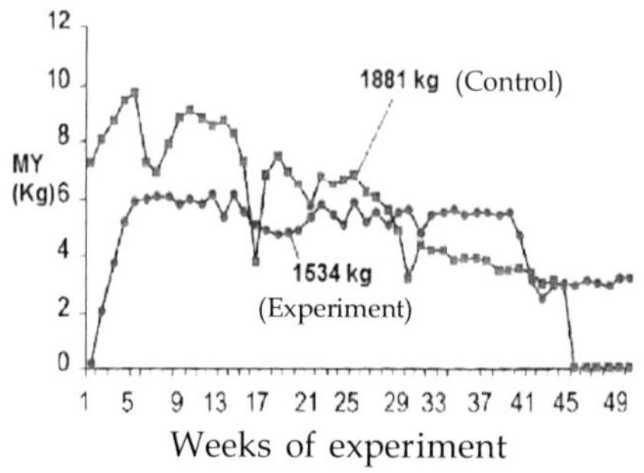

Figure 1.

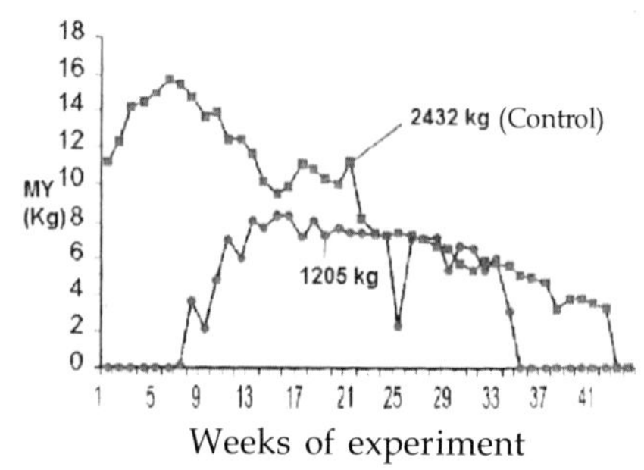

Figure 2.

Milk yield of Buffaloes induced into lactation (control = previous lactation)

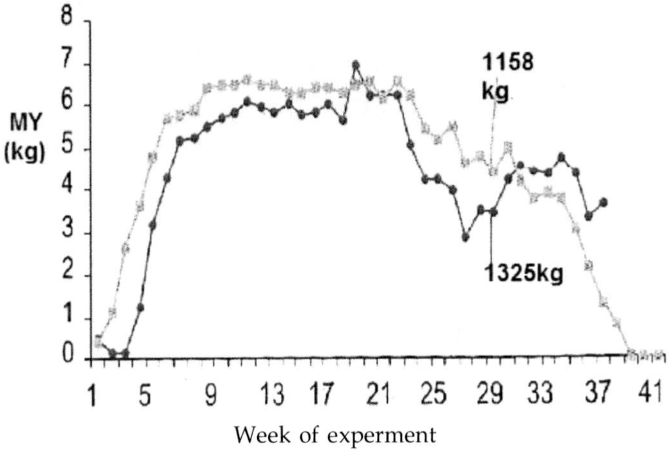

Figure. Lactation curve of primiparopus buffaloes induced into lactation

Chapter-11

Galactopoiesis

The initiation of lactation is a continuous process after the parturition and it continues till peak yield is attained and lactation is established. Galactopoeisis is referred as the maintenance of lactation or milk secretion. Following key factors are responsible for the maintenance of lactation.

i) Synthesis and secretion of milk

ii) Removal of milk

iii) Adequate release and action of galactopoietic hormones

The synthesis and secretion of milk are closely related with each other. Milk synthesis is impaired if milk is not removed from the udder at the time of milking.Growth hormone, prolactin, thyroid hormone, insulin and adrenal corticoids play an important role in milk secretion in lactating animals; however their role differ in different species. The word galactopoiesis is frequently used to indicate enhancement of lactation in dairy animals because of the role of galactopoietic hormones in milk production.

The effect of any substance or hormones as a galactopoietic agent could be known by two methods.

1. Firstly by suppressing plasma concentration of any hormone under study and measure the effect on milk production and composition. The decline in milk yield indicates that hormone is required for maintenance of lactation, although effect may vary depending on the species, stage of lactation and parity.
2. The exogenous administration of precise amount of any hormone during lactation may enhance milk production which indicates that the said hormone is rate limiting in milk secretion and hence it is referred as a galctopoietic hormone. Besides hormones, many non-hormonal preparations and herbal products like shatavari, guduchi,

protected choline chloride, protected amino acids or prill fat have been either fed orally or intra-ruminally to augment milk production in cows, buffaloes and are referred to as a *galactagogue* substances.

Mammary gland is made up of many epithelial cells and alveoli which are in different functional states during different stages of lactation at any time. Mammary gland is not in a static stage during lactation in most species because of this reason. The dynamic changes that occur in the mammary glands during lactation have been studied extensively in goats. Immediately after parturition, milk yield starts increasing and peak yield is achieved around 45 days of lactation in cows and buffaloes. Few animals may achieve peak yield at a very early stage (25-30 days postpartum) and some may take as long as 80-100 days to attain peak yield. After this, milk production is static and maintained for a certain period of time (persistency) and then starts declining with advancement of lactation. The pictorial variation in milk yield during different weeks of lactation is known as 'Lactation curve'. The standard length of lactation is 305 and 150 days in large and small ruminants. The increase in milk yield in early lactation is caused by;

- Increasing numbers of epithelial cells leading to a mammary growth of 10%.
- Increased rate of milk secretion/cell.

However, factors like nutrient availability, metabolic state of animal, management and environment influence milk yield at all stages of lactation. These effects are more pronounced in ascending phase of lactation, peak yield and declining phase of lactation. During late pregnancy programmed cell death, called apoptosis occurs which causes decline in milk secretion. Therefore; milk production during lactation can be augmented by maintaining;

- Number of Alveolar cells,
- Synthetic activity per mammary cell
- Efficacy of milk ejection reflex
- Use of galactagogue substances and
- Balance feeding of cows based on milk yield.

The effect of galactopoietic hormones on milk yield will be effective if the milk ejection is complete and milk is removed frequently from the udder. If milk is not removed efficiently, milk synthesis will not persist despite adequate hormonal status. At the same time, lactation is not maintained indefinitely despite frequent removal of milk. Thus milk secretion and its removal are important in order to maintain lactation in dairy animals.

The qualitative changes in milk yield, number of mammary secretory cells and milk yield/epithelial cell have been studied extensively in goats. Mammary DNA increases by 25% during the initial three weeks of lactation in goats, but peak milk production is attained during eight weeks due to continued activity of lactogenic enzymes and increased differentiation of secretory cells beyond the third week of lactation. In dairy cattle, mammary DNA increases in early lactation, but precise timing and the extent of postpartum mammary growth has not been defined. Postpartum mammary growth may be expected only for a short period during early lactation of cows and buffaloes.The changes in mammary cell numbers by growth or by cell death and milk yield per cell are regulated in part by;

i) Galactopoietic hormones (GH,PRL, CORT, Thyroid hormones) and

ii) Local mammary factors

The table gives a summary of work reported by Knight and Peaker (1984) in goats.

Weeks of Lactation	Phase of the Lactation Curve	Milk Yield	Cell Numbers	Yield per Cell
1	Ascending	Increasing	Increasing	
2	Ascending	Increasing	Increasing	
3	Ascending	Increasing	Increasing	Increasing
4	Ascending	Increasing	Static	Increasing
5	Ascending	Increasing	Static	Increasing
6	Ascending	Static		
7	Peak	Static		
8	Peak	Static	Declining	
8 – 11	Peak	Declining	Declining	
11 - 23	Declining	Declining	Declining	
23 - 36	Late lactation, pregnant	Declining	Static	Declining

Hormonal regulation

The maintenance of lactation in ruminant and non-ruminants is regulated by hormones which are released from;

- Pituitary gland (prolactin, GH, ACTH, TSH)
- Ovary (estrogen)
- Adrenal gland (glucocroticoids and mineralo-corticoids)
- Thyroid gland (T_3& T_4)
- Oxytocin (essential for let down of milk) and
- Mammary glands local growth factors

Prolactin

The role of prolactin in the maintenance of lactation in different species has been studied extensively. However, considerable species variation exists in PRL reqauirement for maintenance of lactation. Hypophysectomy of rabbit leads to immediate cessation of lactation and exogenous PRL administration alone restores lactation to normal. Mammary gland of the rabbit is highly sensitive to PRL and it is galactopoietic in the intact lactating rabbit. Prolactin supplementation prevents normal decline in milk yield of rabbit. Thus in rodents, suppression of PRL decreases milk yield upto 50%. In rabbit, PRL inhibition causes complete failure of lactation. In the hypox. rat- PRL alone does not restore lactation quantitatively to pre-hypox. levels. Administration of PRL and glucocorticoid restore lactation to normal level in hypox. rats. Administration of GH, PRL and glucocorticoids improves lactation performance. High doses of exogenous prolactin stimulate milk secretion in rats by increasing metabolism of the mammary epithelial tissue during early lactation.

In many non-ruminants, suppression of blood PRL concentrations by ergot alkaloids such as bromocryptine reduce lactation performance. Administration of L-DOPA which also inhibits PRL secretion from the pituitary reduces milk yield, although L-DOPA also inhibits milk ejection. Injection of antisera to PRL receptors can inhibit PRL binding in rat mammary gland. This inhibits PRL-induced casein synthesis and milk yield is decreased. Thus role and importance of PRL in maintaining lactation in non- ruminants is well established.

Suppression of PRL in cows and buffaloes by ergot alkaloids or bromocryptine has minimal effects on milk yield. Administration of single injection of bromocryptine @100ug/kg body wt. during early lactation in Murrah buffaloes does not influence yield and composition of milk which suggest that PRL has no role in milk secretion once lactation is fully established. A small quantity of circulating plasma PRL is probably sufficient to maintain lactation after peak lactation. However precise role of PRL in ruminant lactation needs to be elucidated further.

Bromocryptine treatment markedly reduces milk yield in lactating ewe. Mammary uptake of prolactin is highest during milking or after injection of TRH. Similar information is warranted in cattle and buffaloes. Prolactin hormone is bound to the membranes of rough endoplasmic reticulum, Golgi and secretory vesicles and secreted in milk but its physiological functions in milk are unknown. Prolactin is required to maintain lactation during all stages of lactation in goats. Administration of bromocryptine @5mg/d during early and mid lactation decreased plasma prolactin level to non-detectable levels concomitant to decrease in milk yields, protein and lactose contents. The administration of ACTH, GH, T_3 and insulin restored milk production in goats with depressed lactation.

Factors that affects release of PRL

1. Photoperiod
2. Injection of TRH
3. Stress
4. Climate
5. Hypophysectomy/ovariectomy/ adrenalectomy
6. Milking by hand or machine

Use of drugs such as TRH and tranquilizers like reserpine stimulate secretion of prolactin and leads to small increases in milk yields in cattle and women. TRH also release GH and thyroxine hormone and its effect could be due to the combination of hormones.

The number of PRLreceptors is affected by the absence of specific hormones as given below.

Treatment	Decline in PRL receptors in rat mammary tissue
Ovariectomy	59%
Adrenalectomy	45%
Hypophysectomy	35%

Role of milking stimulus on prolactin release

Milking by hand or machine and the calf suckling stimulus causes an immediate increase in concentration of PRL in early lactation in different species. Milking or nursing causes 3 folds increase in PRL release than in non-nursing rats due to decreased release of prolactin inhibiting factor (PIF) from hypothalamus. The suckling induced surge of PRL is small as compared to the peripartum surge of PRL associated with lactogenesis. In dairy cows PRL is not correlated with the milk yield but a correlation between milk yield and PRL levels 5 minutes post milking have been found. Milking-induced PRL surge may last for 30 to 35 minutes post-milking in comparison to oxytocin surge which lasts about 5 to 10 minutes. Milking or suckling induced PRL release declines with advancement of lactation. Stimuli like milking, handling of animal, ambient temperature and photoperiod can alter PRL levels.

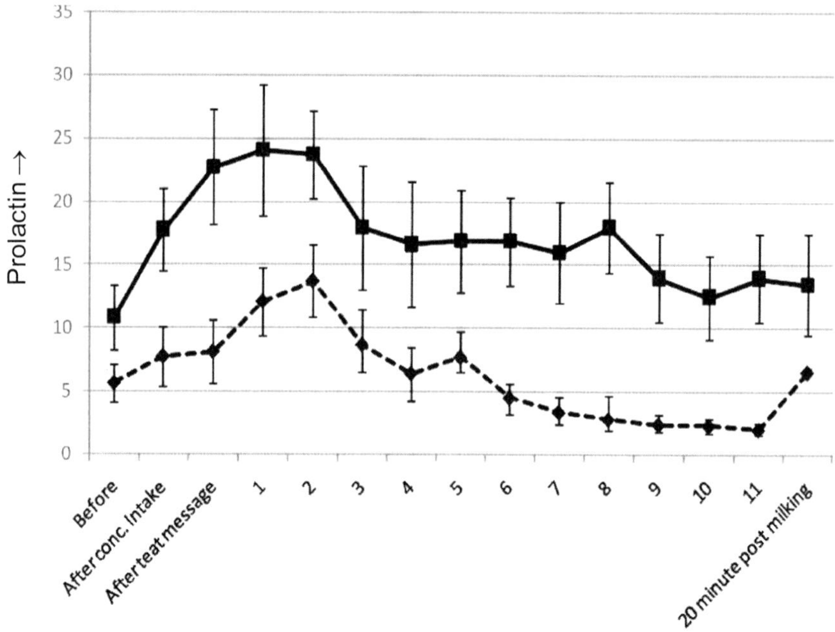

Figure. Effect of hand (■) and machine milking (•) on plasma prolactin (ng/ml) in buffaloes

Effect of photoperiod

Increase in ambient temperature and day length increase blood PRL concentrations although this response lags a few days behind the change in day-length. Blood PRL concentrations also respond to many stress stimuli. Due to these reasons great care should be taken while collecting blood samples for biological studies. Photoperiod induces PRL secretion in cows, buffaloes and goats. Lactating cows given exposure of 16 hr. of light daily produce more milk yields by about 10% during the fall and winter season due to increased feed intake.

Growth hormone

Growth hormone or somatotropin has a molecular weight of 46,000. Somatotropin is a protein hormone with essentially the same structure and biological activity than GH. Bovine growth hormone (bGH) is produced and secreted by cells of the anterior pituitary gland. The mature form of bGH is a single chain of polypeptide containing 191 amino acids and has structural homology with human (63 %) and ovine hormone (97 %). Nursing release growth hormone in rats but in cows, available reports indicate a non-significant rise in GH levels. Plasma GH levels increase with increase in milk yield and decline gradually after peak lactation in ruminants. There is an increased capacity of anterior pituitary gland to release more growth hormone coinciding with high milk secretion. In women the GH concentration in lactating and non-lactating state remains similar.

Nursing causes increased release of GH from the pituitary gland in rats and goats but GH release during milking is not clear. Blood GH levels are positively correlated with milk yield in ruminants and decreases with advancement of lactation when yields decline. The release of GH from the pituitary in response to TRH administration also decreases with advancing lactation. Thus role of growth hormone as a predominant galactopoietic hormone is well established in ruminants. The role of GH in lactation is species specific.

- GH administration has little effect on established lactation in rats.
- GH is galactopoietic in cows and buffaloes.
- GH is necessary to maintain lactation in hypophysectomized lactating goats.
- Prolactin and growth hormonesare required for galactopoiesis in lactating sheep.

Now a day's recombinant bovine Somatotropin (rBST) is produced in large scale by genetically engineering bacteria.

GH has two distinct effects

- **Direct effect:** GH binds with its receptor on target fat cells or adipocytes and stimulates them to break down into triglyceride and suppresses their ability to take up and accumulate circulating lipids.
- **Indirect effect:** GH is mediated primarily by production of insulin like growth factor like IGF-I/IGF-II hormone from the liver and other tissues.

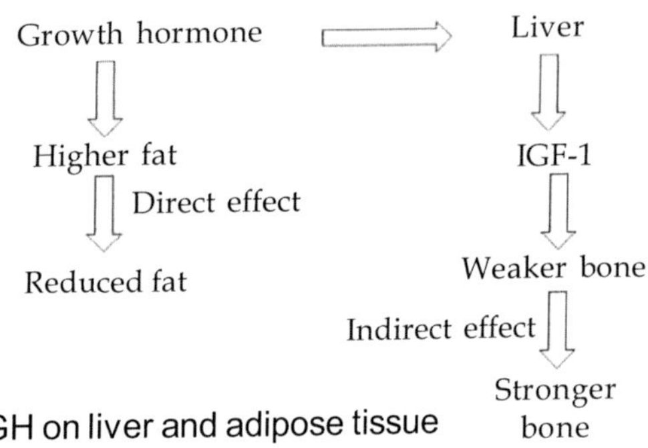

Figure. Effect of GH on liver and adipose tissue

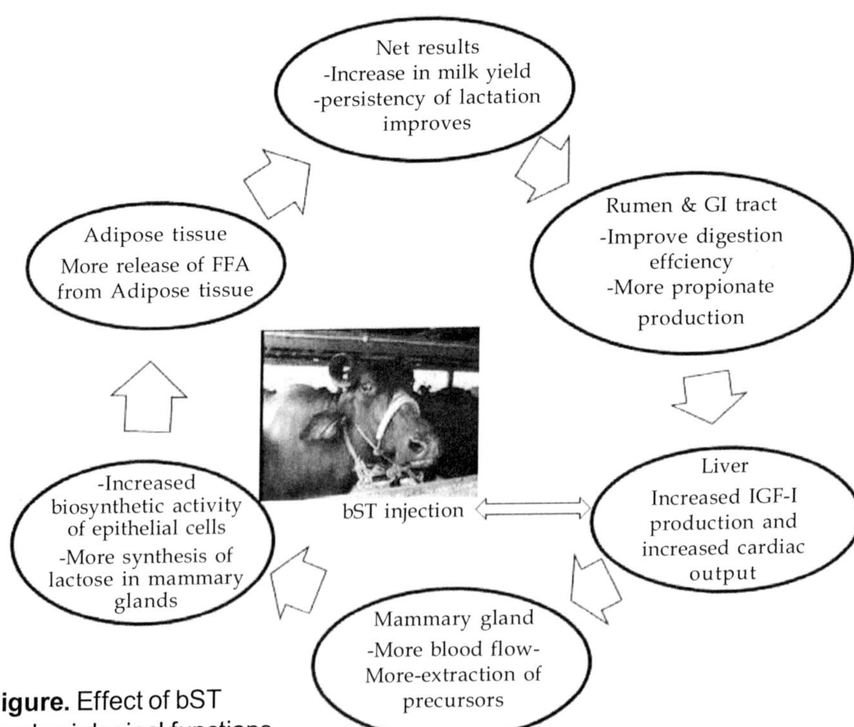

Figure. Effect of bST on physiological functions

Mode of action of bovine somatotropin in ruminants

Milk yield of crossbred Holstein cattle decreases rapidly concomitant to reduction in endogenous growth hormone level and mammary blood flow during lactation. Exogenous bST exert its effect on mammary function to stimulate milk secretion by increasing mammary blood flow and nutrients uptake. An increase in the circulating levels of growth hormone either by subcutaneous injection or daily injections of bST results in increased milk yield in cows and buffaloes by a mechanism without involving the direct action of GH on the udder. GH receptors are not present in the bovine mammary glands and its effects are mediated through IGF-I hormone. Many cells of bovine mammary glands, such as fibroplasts, adipocytes, T-lymophocytes and smooth muscle cells have been shown to possess GH receptors. Bovine somatotropin treatment increases milk production in cows and buffaloes within a lag period of 24 hours by 15-20% in early to mid-lactation and up to 40% during late-lactation.Daily administration of 25 mg/d and 50 mg/d rBST *i.m.;* and slow release formulation of rBST @160 mg/14 d, 320mg/14 d and 500 mg/14 or 30 day,*s/c.* is effiective in increasing the milk production of dairy cows and buffaloes. The release of GH from the injection site is very crucial as it determines the response of rBST on milk yield. If injections are not truly subcutaneous, the response of treatment on milk yield between the animals varies. The rBST treatment results in coordinated changes in tissues and physiological processes that support the increased synthesis of lactose, fat, and protein in the mammary gland. GH treatments improve persistency of lactation and the animals produce more milk for more time. rBST could be given to lactating cows after attaining the peak yield to improve the persistency of lactation and conception rate.

Feed intake of bST treated cows does not increase in short term studies but an increase in DMI (6 to 8%/day) occurs during long term treatment to support the demand of mammary gland for increased milk production. Therefore, such animals need to be given energy rich feed to avoid losses in body weight. GH treatment improves productive efficiency of dairy animals. Milk composition (fat, protein, calcium and lactose) is influenced by bST treatment only when the animals are in negative energy balance.

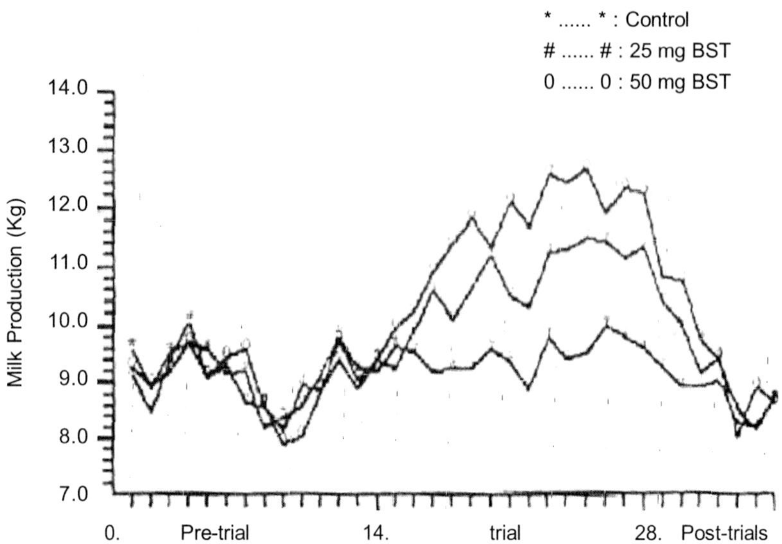

Figure. Effect of daily injection of rBST on milk production of Murrah buffaloes

Table. Concentrations of hormones in plasma of Holsteins injected prepartum with excipient or bST.

Hrmone	Group[1]	Before		Injection phase During[2]		After[3]	
		LSM	SEM	LSM	SEM	LSM	SEM
				(mg/ml)			
Insulla	Control4	1.38	.04	1.35	.04	1.39	.05
	Treated	1.35	.04	1.30	.04	1.39	.05
Triiodothysomine	Control	.46	.09	.47	.04	.65	.05
	Treated	.51	.09	.50	.04	.64	.05
Thyroxine	Control	29.0	3.0	24.9	2.2	25.9	2.6
	Treated	33.2	2.9	25.9	2.2	25.2	2.6
Cortisol	Control	15.17	2.23	13.36	1.06*	11.56	2.11
	Treated	18.36	2.49	9.64	1.18	13.72	2.40
Prolactin	Control	6.03	.47	9.00	1.5	7.35	1.8
	Treated	8.75	.47	8.27	8.5	11.73	1.8
Somatotropin	Control	3.46	.63	4.71	1.01**	6.47	1.02
	Treated	3.28	.71	13.35	1.13	5.90	1.11
Insulin-like growth	Control	51.46	3.64*	48.83	6.35	49.57	6.94
factor-I	Treated	64.35	4.07	55.96	7.2	35.81	7.50

[1] Control heifers and dry cows received sodium bicarbecate excipient, and treated group received bST (25 mg/d) for 14 consocutive d.

[2] Adjusted for before treatment values.

[3] Adjusted for both before and during treatment values.

[4] Samples analyzed for control and treated groups before, during, and after injection were 21 and 22; 23 and 26; and 80 and 79 within each hormone analyzed. Means for control and treatment groups within phase were compared.

op < .05 oop < .001

Effect on animal health

Conflicting reports are available regarding the effect of rBST on animal health and reproduction.

According to few reports, there are no adverse effects of rBST on health of animals, reproduction, and parturition, health of neonate and mastitis incidence. But few findings indicate that rBST treatment causes nearly 25% increase in the risk of clinical mastitis, a 40% reduction in fertility, 55% increased risk of developing clinical signs of lameness, a decrease in body condition score even though there was an increase in dry matter intake. European Union Commission stated that the use of rBST substantially increase health problems like foot problems, mastitis, injection site reactions, impinged on the welfare of the animals and reproductive disorders in cows. The report concluded that rBST should not be used. Many research works in this direction suggest that such problems are normally associated with high milk producing animals and not necessarily caused by bST administration.

Human health concern

Use of BST is controversial primarily due to concerns over potential harmful effects on animal and human health. Food products made from rBST treated cows are considered to be safe for human consumption and no significant difference exists between milk derived from rBST-treated and non-rBST-treated cows. The FDA reported bovine GH to be biologically inactive when consumed by humans and found no biological distinction between rBST and BST. In 1990, an independent panel convened by the National Institute of Health supported the FDA opinion that milk and meat from cows supplemented with rBST are safe for human consumption.

Plasma GH level increase in rBST administered animals which may appear in the milk also. Some studies have shown that milk composition of rbST treated (10ppb) cows is similar to the milk of non treated cows. The research findings also suggest that about 90% of milk GH is destroyed by pasteurization and rest is digested in the gastrointestinal tract of animals as another protein. GH shows species-specificity,If it persists and enters the blood stream it would not be active in humans. Further, milk IGF-1 level remains within normal range in the treated cows.

IGF-1

IGF-I hormone is a single chain peptides of 70 amino acids, synthesized mainly in the liver and other tissues. It has been detected in the milk from many species. The increase in milk yield coincides with increased concentrations of plasma and milk IGF-I in the treated animals. IGF-I level increase by 2-5 ng/ml after rBST injection in cows. The normal values of IGF-I have been reported between 3 to 10ng/ml in cow milk and 1-3 ng/ml in human milk. IGF-I is produced normally and is present in saliva, pancreatic juice, secretion from intestinal mucosa, liver,extrahepatic tissues and mammary gland. Many views have been put to explain that milk of GH/ IGF-I treated cows does not have any adverse effect on human helath. i) The amount of IGF-I consumed daily from milk products is minute as compared to natural endogenous production in human body ii) IGF-I cannot be absorbed through stomach or intestineand subjected to proteolysis during intestinal passage and iii) small amounts absorbed by intestine will contribute <0.06% of the total daily IGF-I production. An infusion of IGF-I stimulates blood flow to the mammary glands and increases milk production. Administration of rBST in lactating cows and buffaloes increases bovine IGF-1 in milk, a structure that is identical in cows and humans. It has been found that only difference between milk from supplemented and un-supplemented cattle is the amount of IGF-1 however elevated levels are similar to levels found in milk from untreated cows. Further, amount of IGF-1 consumed in milk is negligible as compared to amount produced in the body. Available lierature suggest that higher IGF-1 level being resistant to pasteurization may lead to increased risk of breast, colon, and prostate cancer.

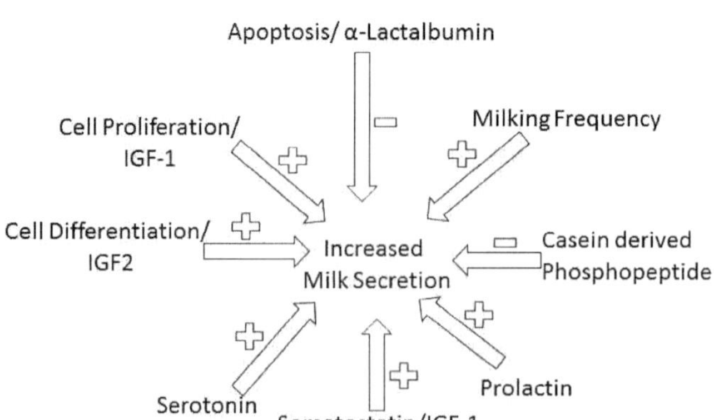

Figure. Factors affecting galactopoiesis in dairy animals

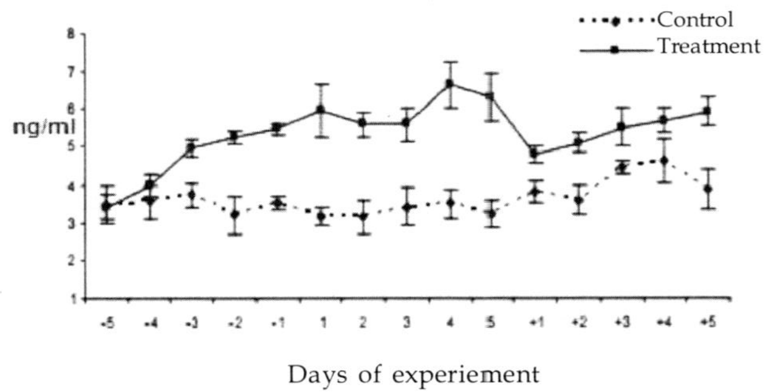

Plasma GH levels in Murrah buffaloes administered rBST during early lactation

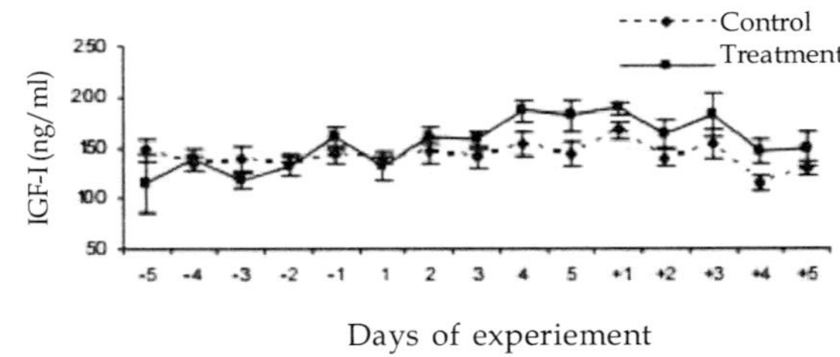

Plasma IGF-I levels in Murrah buffaloes administered rBST during early lactation

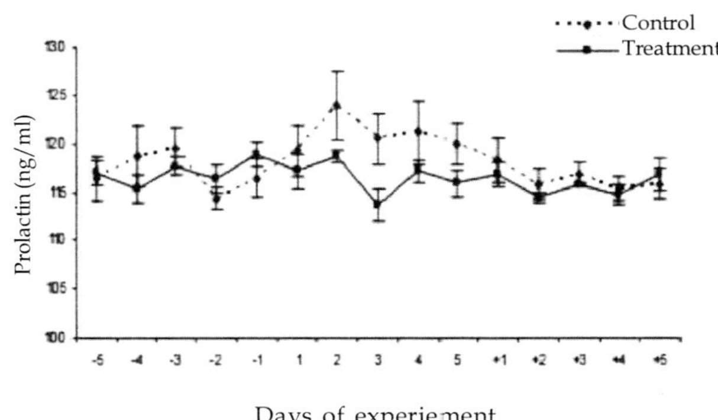

Plasma prolactin levels in Murrah buffaloes administered rBST during early lactation

Milk IGF-I concentration before, during and after the administration of rBST.

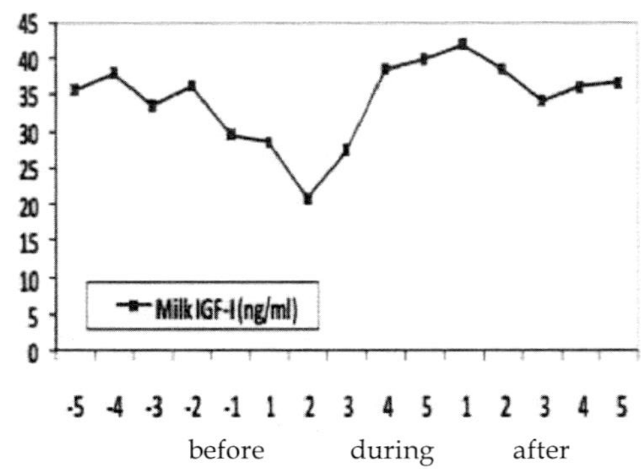

Adrenal hormones

Adrenalectomy impairs milk secretion; reduce enzymatic function and casein mRNA synthesis in laboratory animals. Administration of either mineralo or glucocorticoids partially restores milk yield. Supplementation of both mineralocorticoids and glucocorticoids restore milk yield fully. This fact suggests that adrenal steroids are necessary for the maintenance of lactation. Adrenalectomy causes impairement of electrolyte, protein and carbohydrate metabolism. However, their role in ruminant lactation is less clear.

Injection of cortisone, corticosterone or cortisol acetate stimulate lactation performance by 12-27% in lactating rat, but administration of glucocorticoids inhibit lactation in high doses.

Lower doses stimulate milk yield in early lactation and preventsthe expected decline in milk yield in late lactation. In adrenalectomized rat, milk secretion is impaired and casein mRNA levels are decreased by 85-92%. Cortisol administration reverses the changes. Adrenalectomy-ovariectomy stops lactation completely.

Adrenal corticoid content is highly correlated with mammary nucleic acid content during lactation. Blood corticoids levels remain similar during lactation but fluctuate during different seasons. The concentration of corticoids declines due to their binding with corticoid binding globulin (CBG) during early lactation. Blood concentration of CBG declines during early lactation and increases during later part of lactation in laboratory animals, but there is no change in CBG during lactation in cows.

Injection of glucocorticoids decrease milk yield temporarily due to the reduced uptake of glucose by mammary glands in cows. In ruminants the low dose of glucocorticoids is crucial as some workers have found an increase in milk yield of early lactating cows. Glucocorticoids are released acutely in response to milking stimulus in cows, buffaloes, sheep, goat and rat. The tactile induced release of cortisol is maintained as lactation progresses, as cows do not lose their ability to release glucocorticoids. However suckling induced increase of glucocorticoids decline with advancement of lactation in rats and controls the rate of milk secretion. Adrenal secretions are rate limiting during advanced lactation in rat and highly correlated with DNA during lactation. Mammary glands of pregnant goats remove about 2.8% of the total cortisol and have about 7500 specific binding sites for cortisol. The mammary uptake of cortisol is not affected by testosterone and estrogen but inhibited by progesterone. The number of molecules of cortisol binding to each mammary cell depends on physiological state of a lactating animal. During prepartum period the number of cortisol molecule binding to the epithelial cell is 520 which increase during lactating state (1242), however, in virgin and dry state the number of molecule binding to epithelial cells is less (387 vs.307). Corticoids are not rate limiting to milk yield in cows and buffaloes, but they are not unnecessary for lactation.

The concentration of adrenal steroid is markedly influenced by the climate and ambient temperature. Cortiosl secretion is influenced by the extremes of summer and winter seasons in ruminants. At low ambient temperature (15°C) high producing cows have greater concentrations of glucocorticoids than the low producers. At high temperature (>30°C) the high producing cows secrete less glucocorticoids than the low producers. Due to this reason high producers are less persistent than the low milk producers during hot-weather conditions. The concentration of glucocorticoids fluctuates during lactation but physiological significance of corticoids secretion into milk remains to be investigated.

Thyroid hormones

Thyroid hormones (T_3 and T_4) are essential for maximal secretion of milk. This fact is clear from the experiment in which thyroid gland is removed and its effects on milk production are observed.

- Thyroidectomy or irradiating the thyroid gland by ingesting radioactive iodine in cattle results in decreased milk yield. Injection of thyroid hormone in cattle for 7 weeks at 25% above the normal thyroid secretion rate results in increased milk yield by 27%. However, thyroid hormone administration at 150% for 7 or more weeks has little or no effect on milk yield.

In cattle, milking stimulus does not release thyroid hormone. Also there is no change in thyroxine binding globulin (TBG) during lactation. After parturition the dairy cattle and buffaloes are under very high metabolic demands due to increasing trend of milk in early lactation. So there is an inverse relationship between a cow's milk yield and blood levels of thyroid hormones in early lactation. Keeping this fact in mind feeding of iodinated casein or thyroprotein is being practiced to augment milk production of dairy animals. Providing extra thyroxine during lactation explains the galactopoietic effect of thyroxine in dairy cattle. Feeding of thyroprotein (iodinated casein) increases milk yield by 10 and 15-20% in early and late lactation, but effect on milk yield lasts only for 2-4 months in cows. After withdrawal of treatment subsequent milk yields are below normal. Extra feed must be provided during the feeding of thyroprotein and it should be fed only when cows are gaining body weight. Considering the economics, there is no net benefit of feeding thyroprotein over the entire lactation length. The transient increase in milk yield in thyroprotein fed cows occurs only when feed intake is increased.

Mechanisms of thyroid hormone action

The thyroid secretions strongly influence milk synthesis though some milk secretion will continue in the absence of thyroid hormones. Thyroid stimulating hormone (TSH) is secreted by the anterior pituitary gland which stimulates secretion of thyroid hormones from thyroid gland. The primary thyroid hormone produced in thyroid gland is thyroxine (3,5,3',5'-tetraiodothyronine; or T_4). The T_4 is an alanine molecule with a tyrosyl ring and a phenolic ring, each of which is iodinated at the 3 and 5 and 3' and 5' carbon positions, respectively. However, T_4 has relatively low affinity for thyroid hormone receptors in target tissues and is considered a prohormone requiring further modification to achieve full activity. The major biologically active form of thyroid hormone is T_3 (3,5,3'-tri-iodothyronine). Deiodination of T_4 can occur in the thyroid gland or in the various target tissues. The following specific deiodinase enzymes have been identified, each belonging to a family of selenocysteine-containing enzymes.

Type I deiodinase is found predominantly in the liver, kidney, thyroid, skeletal muscle, heart, lung, intestine and mammary gland in the rat. It can catalyze either 5'- or 5-monodeiodination. The 5'-deiodination removes an iodine from the outer phenolic ring, resulting in formation of the active T_3 (3, 5, 3′-tri-iodothyronine), while 5-deiodination removes an iodine from the inner tyrosyl ring, resulting in the inactive reverse T_3 (3,3',5'-tri-iodothyronine). Mammary gland of the rat has Type I deiodinase activity. Type II deiodinase is found in central nervous system (cerebral cortex, cerebellum, and hypothalamus), pituitary, and brown adipose tissue (BAT). Type II deiodinase catalyzes only removal of the 5'-iodine. Therefore, type II deiodinase will convert T_4 to T_3 while rT_3 is converted to the inactive T_2 (3,3'-di-iodothyronine). Type II deiodinase activity is present in the cow and mouse mammary glands. Sow's mammary gland possesses both Type I and II deiodinase activity.

Type III deiodinase has 5-deiodinase activity and therefore converts active T_4 or T_3 to inactive rT_3 or T_2, respectively. Type III deiodinase is found in cerebral cortex and skin, but also in several tissues of the fetus. It may be involved in metabolizing active thyroid hormone in the fetus to protect the fetal brain and other tissues from exposure to high levels of thyroid hormones.

There is a considerable species varation for the type of deiodinase present in the mammary gland. Deiodination of thyroid hormones by peripheral tissues, including the mammary gland, plays a primary role in regulating thyroid hormone homeostasis, and therefore is indicative of the metabolic state of the animal and of the particular tissue. The high activity of deiodinase in the mammary gland results in more local production of T_3 which in turn stimulates mammary metabolism.The excessive local conversion of T_4 to T_3 in the mammary gland may reduce blood levels of T_4during early lactation in cows and buffaloes. Administration of T_3 bypasses the conversion T_4 to T_3 at the mammary gland level and provides greater T_3 to the gland resulting in enhanced milk yield in cows.

Calcitonin

Calcitonin is released from the thyroid gland in response to high blood calcium levels. Blood calcium concentration is more in lactating animals than non-lactating animals. This hormone does not have a direct role in the maintenance of lactation, but is important in view of the high concentration of calcium secreted in milk. It prevents increase in serum calcium and phosphorus during lactation.

Parathyroid hormone

Removal of parathyroid gland reduces milk yield and blood calcium concentration during lactation. Administration of hormone increases milk yield and calcium concentration. Hypocalcemia induces release of parathyroid hormone which acts in two wasy to increase calcium concentration in blood. i) This hormone converts vitamin D into 25-hydroxy-vitamin-D and then to 1,25-dihydroxy-vitaminD (1,25-OHD). The later stimulate calcium absorption from GI tract. ii) It causes calcium and phosphorous mobilization from the bone.

Therefore, role of parathryroid hormne is important from the point of view of calcium homeostasis and large calcium drain into milk during lactation.

Insulin

The concentration of insulin is low during early lactation and gradually increases in mid and late lactation in cows. Administration of insulin suppresses lactation, while insufficiency of insulin also decreases milk yield. Plasma insulin concentrations are negatively correlated with milk yield. Insulin is important for maintenance of lactation as mammary uptake of insulin is associated with uptake of glucose during lactation, but it is not rate limiting.

Estrogen

The role of two major hormones of ovary *i.e.* estrogen and progesterone is very much limited during lactation. Ovariectomy during lactation has little effect on milk secretion while exogenous administration of estrogen inhibits lactation. The inhibitory effect is exerted directly on the mammary gland by the disappearance of myofilaments of myoepithelail cells; thererby interferes with normal process of let-down of milk. A very low dose of estrogen stimulates milk secretion by its effect on galactopoietics hormone (PRL) from the anterior pituitary gland.

Progesterone

Progesterone is anti-lactogenic and its administration does not affect milk yield during lactation due to the less number of progesterone binding sites in lactating mammary tissue and more affinity of progesterone for milk fat than for its receptors. Progesterone is secreted into alveolar lumen along with fat. Due to these reasons the effect of progesterone administration on milk yield does not occur during lactation. Progesterone concentration in milk parallels closely with its blood concentration. That is why milk progesterone concentration is used to diagnose pregnancy on day 21 post-insemination. The elevated plasma progesterone levels in milk indicate pregnancy with 70% accuracy. In case of low progesterone concentration the animals are confirmed as non-pregnant with 90 % accuracy.

Placental lactogen

Cattle are lactating often and pregnant at the same time, unlike many species. Consequently, placental hormones may affect mammary function. Bovine placental lactogen administration during lactation increase milk yield in dairy cattle though relatively little placental lactogen is released into the mother's blood in cows. The goat generally is non-lactating and pregnant at the same time. In contrast to cows, very high levels of caprine placental lactogen are found in the pregnant goat's blood which has a dramatic effect on mammary development of the goat.

Oxytocin

Oxytocin is required to letdown the milk and stimulates milk secretion. Several experiments using injection of oxytocin in cows indicate that it facilitates faster let-down of milk. Injection of oxytocin in rat during early lactation stimulate milk yield by 13% but a non-significant effect on milk yield have been reported in cows due to the milking of animals immediately after injection. The release of oxytocin is adversely affected by fear, pain, disturbed milking operations, change of milking man and place of milking. The milking operation needs to be carried out within 4-5 minutes either by hand or machine due to a very short half life of oxytocin. However in a congenial environment, the amount of oxytocin released at milking is higher. The release of oxytocin declines with advancement of lactation just like prolactin. Oxytocin maintains the integrity of mammary epithelial cells and the effects may be mediated through the release of prolactin.

Practical exercises on lactation

Average milking rate

Milking rate of dairy cows is an important consideration for the dairyman. It determines the speed with which a cow can be milked, that ultimately affects the number of cows that can be milked by a milker in a unit time. Average milking rate is defined in simple words as the amount of milk drawn from the udder per unit time. It consists of 3 phases- slow stripping, fast milking and the last stripping.

Maximum Milking Rate - It is the highest yield during any interval of milking process and is usually measured in one minute. The maximum milking rate is obtained at first minute of milking.

Factors affecting milking rate are,

1. Teat orifice
2. Internal udder pressure
3. Capacity of the teat meatus
4. Milk yield
5. Breed and inheritance difference.

Exercise 1. Calculating the average milking rate of cows.

Animal	Milking time (sec.)	Milk yield (gm)	Av. Milking rate(gm/sec)
1	175	3000	17.10
2	85	2100	24.70
3	180	2000	11.12

Exercise 2. Dissection of rat's mammary glands

Dissection is carried out to count the number of mammary glands and record the weight of these glands. The rat has six pairs of mammary glands out of which 3 are thoracic, one each is abdominal and two pairs are inguinal glands. A female rat is anesthetized with the help of chloroform and kept on the dissecting tray, with ventral side upwards. The mammary glands are counted to see their positions. An incision is made along the middle of the rat by locating the mammary glands on the inner side of the skin. Mammary glands are flat and embedded in the skin. The mammary glands are clearly visible after removal of subcutaneous tissues. The glands are put on a filter paper for weighing.

Observations on mammary glands.

i) Weight of filter paper = 258 mg

ii) Weight of mammary gland with paper = 290 mg

iii) Weight of mammary gland = 32 mg

Now days, due to animal ethicol point of view, the experiments are carried out with specific models.

Exercise 3. Estimation of residual milk and rate of milk secretion in cows

At first the animal is milked dry. Then 10.I.U. of 1 ml synthetic oxytocin in sterile saline soloution is injected into the jugular vein. After one or two minutes the cow is milked again. The amount of milk obtained is weighed in both cases. The quantity of milk obtained during first milking is reffered to as normal milk where as that obtained after second milking is reffered as residual milk. Total milk can be calculated by adding the quantity of milk obtained in two milkings and residual milk is calculated on the percentage basis. The percentage of residual milk stays same throughout the lactation. Older cows have higher percentage of residual milk than first calf heifers. The percentage of residual milk is higher in low producers than that of high producers. Animals having low percentage of residual milk are preffered for dairying purpose. The residual milk percentage is an inherited characteristic of animals. Hand milking has been shown to reduce the amount of residual milk as compared to machine milking.

Observations

Animal	Qty. of milk	Residual milk	Total milk yield	% Residual after milking milk
3071	1.8 Kg	150 gm	1.95 Kg	7.69
1553	1.9 Kg	400 gm	2.30 Kg	17.39

It is clear from the above observations that animal No. 3071 is better than that 1553, as the former retains less residual milk (7.69%) than the later (17.39%).

The milk secretion rate can be determined by evacuating the udder of the animal with the help of 10 I.U. of synthetic oxytocin injected in the jugular vein at a given time. The animal is milked dry at the next milking and then the udder is evacuated with the help of oxytocin. The time is noted again. The time elapsed between the two injections is calculated. The amount of milk obtained in between the two injections is also recorded to calculate the rate of milk secretion per minute.

Observations

Time of Ist inj.	Time of 2nd injection	Time elapsed	Amount of milk	Milk secretion rate
6.30 A.M.	2.45	495 min	1.95 Kgs	3.94 gm/min
6.40 A.M.	2.50	490 min	2.30 Kgs	4.69 gm/min

It is obvious that the second cow has more milk secretion rate (4.69 gm/min.) than the first one (3.94 gm/min).

Therefore, total milk yield (Kg) is calucalted by normal milk (Kg) plus residual milk (Kg). The actual milk yield is calculated by subtracting residual milk from the total milk yield. Absolute milk secretion rate can be obtained by dividing actual milk yield by time interval. Similarly apparent milk secretion rate can be calculated while dividing the total milk yield by time interval. Residual milk, apparent milk secretion rate and absolute milk secretion rate can be interpreted from the following exercise.

Exercise 4. In a milking management, the cows were milked at 6, 7 and 11 hourly intervals, and at normal milking they produced 4, 4.5 and 7 Kgs. of milk. As an inherent quality,cow retained 15% residual mik. Calculate the absolute amount and total amount of milk and also calculate the apparent and absolute milk secretion rate.

Solution

Milk obtained at normal milking (Kg)	Residual milk (absolute, kg)	Total milk (Kg)	Residual milk (%)	Time interval (hrs)
4.0	0.71	4.71	15	6
4.5	0.79	5.29	15	7
7.0	1.23	8.23	15	11

When residual milk is 15%, then the amount of normal milk = 100-15 = 85 Kg.

Since 85 Kg of normal milk has a residual milk of 15 Kg therefore, 4 Kg of normal milk will have a residual milk equal to- 15/85 multiplied by 4 which is 0.71 kg at 6 hrs interval.

So, the total milk is = 4+0.71 = 4.71 Kg

Similarly at 7 hrs interval the residual milk = 15/85x4.5 = 0.79Kg

And total milk is = 4.5+0.79 = 5.29 Kg

At 11 hrs interval, the residual milk = 15/85x 7 = 1.23 Kg

And total milk yield is = 7+1.23 = 8.23 Kg

Therefore, total milk production at different intervals is given below as-

a) At 6 hr._________4.71 Kg
b) At 7 hr. _________5.29 Kg
c) At 11 hr.________ 8.23 Kg

The apparent milk secretion rate can be calculated as follows-

a) At 6 hr. 4/6= 0.66 Kg/hr.
b) At 7 hr. 4.5/7= 0.64 Kg/hr.
c) At 11 hr. 7/11= 0.636 Kg/hr.

Absolute milk secretion rate can be calculated as follows-

a) At 6 hr. = (4.71- 1.23)/6 = 3.48/6 = 0.58 Kg /hr.
b) At 7 hr. = (5.29- 0.71)/7 = 4.58/7 = 0.654 Kg /hr.
c) At 11 hr. = (8.23- 0.79)/11 = 7.44/11 = 0.676 Kg /hr.

If oxytocin is not injected then the residual milk present is to be omitted and therefore the residual milk of previous period will be added and it is divided by the time interval.

Exercise 5. A dissection of mammary gland is carried out to trace out the arteries and veins in the udder. The udder is cut open through teats, up to the tissue parenchyma and internal structures are exposed.

The arteries are easily recognized by their hardeness and thick wall since these are slightly darker in shade. The protruding part of artery is held with the help of forceps and the tissue is removed around the artery. Similary the vein is also removed which is characterized by softer tissue. The branching of arteries and veins are carefully separated from the parenchyma tissue without cutting them. A sharp longitudinal incision is made along the midline of udder from anterior to posterior between the two adjacent tissues of median suspansary ligament. The two halves of udder are separated out by pulling them apart and cutting. The teat openings are identified and a deep incision is made to open up the teat cistern and gland cistern. Now days, specific models are being used for academic purpare to explain the arterial and venous system.

❑❑❑

Chapter-12

Body Condition Score

Body condition score (BCS) of an animal can be used as an effective management tool for evaluating the energy reserves.The nutritional requirement for a cow can be made throughout the year to obtain a desirable BCS. Lactating cows and buffaloes that are too lean or obese can have problems of repeat breeding, health disorders, calving problems and excessive feed costs. Many workers have developed BCS system to estimate average body condition of cows. BCS can be determined by a relative score based on an evaluation of fat deposits in relation to skeletal features. Animals can be assessed by visual observation from a short distance. However, manual palpation with visual observation adds to more accuracy. There is a strong correlation between the scoring system and actual fat deposition in the animal.

Fat deposition sites in cows

Body condition score can be used to achieve optimum body condition at calving which helps in maximizing the reproductive and productive efficiency of the herd. It is prudent to evaluate BCS after every 90 to 120 days, at 30 days prior to breeding, 90 days post-breeding, weaning and 100 days prior to calving and at the time of calving. Many factors influence BCS of the animals throughout the year. Postpartum cows have high nutritional requirements for lactation and thus prone to loose their body weights. The cow prepares for rebreeding during this time. Normal reproductive function requires a certain level of fat reserves. Mature cows of all breeds and crosses should have a BCS of 5 at calving to achieve adequate reproductive functions in the subsequent breeding season. The transition from gestation to lactation is often a perilous period in the lactation cycle of the dairy cow. The events occurring in this period are probably among the most significant factors that predispose dairy cows to condition of poor health. Most common diseases that arise in dairy cows occur during periparturient period. The incidence of dystocia, retained foetal membranes, fatty liver, ketosis, displaced abomasum and milk fever are influenced by BCS. It has been shown that dairy cows recovering from milk fever are eight times more likely to develop mastitis in the following lactation and may have a reduced immune competence, along with slower uterine involution. There are several criteria which can help us to monitor energy balance in the animals. However,these criteria per se may not be the perfect predictors of energy balance. BCS is important for ;

- Monitoring the health management of animals in the herd
- Treating metabolic disorders like milk fever and ketosis at calving
- For assessing metabolic and oxidative stress during summer
- For knowing the production ability of cows
- Evaluating ideal health during dry period and calving with optimum BCS of 3.5-4.5

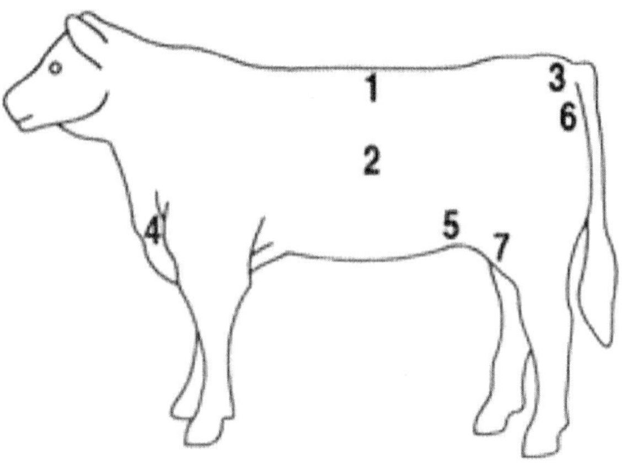

Method of recording BCS

BCS of a cow or buffalo can be evaluated by observing the fat deposition on the backbone, loin and rump areas. Since the pin bone, hip bone, the top of the backbone and ends of the short ribs do not have muscular tissue covering them, therefore a combination of skin and fat deposits are visible in these areas. Press the fingertips against the backbone, pin bone and hip bone. Grip the loin of the cow where the short ribs project from the backbone, just ahead of the hips, with fingers on top of the loin and the thumb curved around the ends of the short ribs. The pressure of fingertip provides a good indication of the fat cover. Different methods have been developed however BCS can be judged with the following simple score of 5 points.

BCS	Status of body
1.	Very thin cow with no fat reservesends of ribs sharp, loin sharp, hook and pin bones are sharp, anal area receded, vulva appears prominent.
2.	Thin cow, ends of the short ribs can be felt, less prominent, area around the anus is less sunken and the vulva less prominent.
3.	Cow in average body condition, short ribs can be felt by applying slight hand pressure, backbone is a rounded ridge and hook and pin bones are round and smooth, anal area is filled but fat deposit
4.	A cow in heavy condition, short ribs can be felt only with firm pressure, hook bones are smooth and flat, area around the pin bones show little fat deposits.
5.	A fat animal. The bone structure of the topline, hook and pin bones and the short ribs is not visible, distinct fat deposits around the tailbone and over the ribs, Over fatty cow or buffalo with fat deposits on thigh and body.

Negative energy balance and its impact on animal productivity

Dairy cows usually suffer from a negative energy balance (NEBAL) in periparturient period due to increased energy requirements and physio-endocrinological changes. NEBAL mobilizes the body energy reserves like glycogen, fat and protein to compensate for their energy needs. Increased lipolysis causes an elevation of non-esterified fatty acids (NEFA) in the blood which results in fatty liver and ketosis. Combined effect of NEBAL, increased lipolysis and fatty liver is associated with suboptimal milk production, poor health and reproductive disorders in postparturient dairy animals. The dairy cows raised in smaller farms have low blood glucose concentration after calving and loose their BCS during the first month of lactation. More NEFA are taken up by the liver as concentration of NEFA in blood increases around calving or early lactation. Ruminants have low capacity for the synthesis and secretion of very-low density lipoproteins

(VLDL) to export triglyceride from the liver but have a similar capacity to reconvert NEFA to triglyceride. Since triglycerides production increases at the time of calving thereofore, the cows fed on typical diets during the dry and transition periods have an increased concentration of triglyceride in the liver on day-1 after calving. Fatty liver develops if NEFA uptake by the liver is excessive. NEBAL and carbohydrate insufficiency in the liver after calving leads to increased production of ketone bodies or ketosis. The NEBAL and rate of mobilization of body reserves results in decreased fertility by delaying the ovarian activity, reduced number of estrous cycles and lower conception rate. NEBAL acts similarly to underfed animals and leads to delayed ovarian activity by impinging on pulsatile secretion of LH. Lower availability of glucose and insulin may also decrease LH pulsatility and limit ovarian responsiveness to gonadotropins.

Table. Ideal BCS during different stages of life in cows and buffaloes

S.No.	Stage of animal	BCS	Remarks
1.	Time of parturition	3 - 4	BCS less than 3 is indicative of mal-nutrition which may affect the coming lactation
2.	Early lactation	3	BCS less than 3 may lead to negative energy balance and may lead to further drop of BCS
3.	Mid-lactation	3	Feed enough to the animals to maintain maximum milk production during this time
4.	Late lactation	3-4	Do not feed more to exceed BCS beyond 4, Cows get ready for the next lactation
5.	Dry period	3-4	Do not feed more to go beyond 4
6.	Heifers	3	If less than 3, the animal may face difficulties in breeding; if more than 3 it may lead to poor milk production during lactation

❑❑❑

Chapter-13

Milk Borne System of Down Regulating the Milk Secretion

As we discussed in earlier chapters, the synthesis of milk is a continual process in the epithelial cells of mammary gland. The remoaval of milk enhances the synthesis of its constituents in the mammary gland. However, if milk removal is impaired then local mammary factors like Feed Back Inhibitors of lactation (FIL) inhibits the rate of milk synthesis and secretion in an epithelial cell. Tissue-explant bioassay studies revealed goat's milk whey proteins (not caseins) inhibit synthesis of casein and lactose in a dose-dependent manner but this inhibition is reversible. Similar inhibitory whey proteins have also been identified in milk of goat, cow and humans. The autocrine mechanism of milk secretion is activated by contact of milk FIL with epithelial cells. The FIL is not activated unless it comes in contact of epithelial cells. The intensity of inhibition is more when milk FIL is more in lumen of alveoli. It has been found that morphology of the Golgi and endoplasmic reticulum are markedly altered and the protein secretion reduces by about 50% within 1h of addition of FIL to the tissue cultures and the secretion rate is restored within 1h of removal of FIL.

Feedback inhibitors of lactation

In many species feedback inhibitor of lactation (FIL) regulates milk secretion. FIL, a milk whey protein (7600 kDa molecular weight) have been measured in milk. FIL is secreted by the epithelial cells during normal course of milk secretion. It inhibits milk synthesis and secretion when its own concentration rises in alveolar lumen. Frequent removal of milk from the mammary gland minimizes local inhibitory effects of FIL and increase milk secretion. The exact mechanism of action of FIL is unknown, but *in-vitro* studies indicate that milk secretion stops as FIL increase. FIL accumulation causes;

- Reduced secretory rate and key enzymes activity in mammary cells,
- Stimulates intracellular degradation of newly synthesized casein mRNA
- Reduces prolactin receptor numbers on the cells and
- Probably inhibit differentiation of mammary cell function.

Thus milk secretion process is regulated by a balance between systemic (hormonal) and local (FIL) control. The following changes take place when tactile stimuli are given at each milking.

- Prolactin release is stimulated
- Intra-mammary pressure is relieved and
- FIL is removed from the alveoli

Facors like irregular milking interval, incomplete milking or no milking of animal results in;

- No stimulation of PRL release and
- Acute accumulation of milk in the mammary gland which resuls in:
    - Increased intra-mammary pressure
    - Activation of sympathetic nerves
    - Decreased mammary blood flow
    - Decreased availability of hormones and nutrients to the gland
    - Decreased rate of milk secretion

This interplay between the systemic hormones and local factors (FIL) control milk secretion in the mammary gland.

The mammary gland is under the influence of the systemic factors (hormone) shortly after milking and maximal milk secretion rate is achieved. This gradually slows down with accumulation of milk as local factors (FIL) become dominant. If milk is not removed, then milk secretion rate eventually drop to zero (see figure), however, under normal milking intervals, the secretion rate does not go to zero.

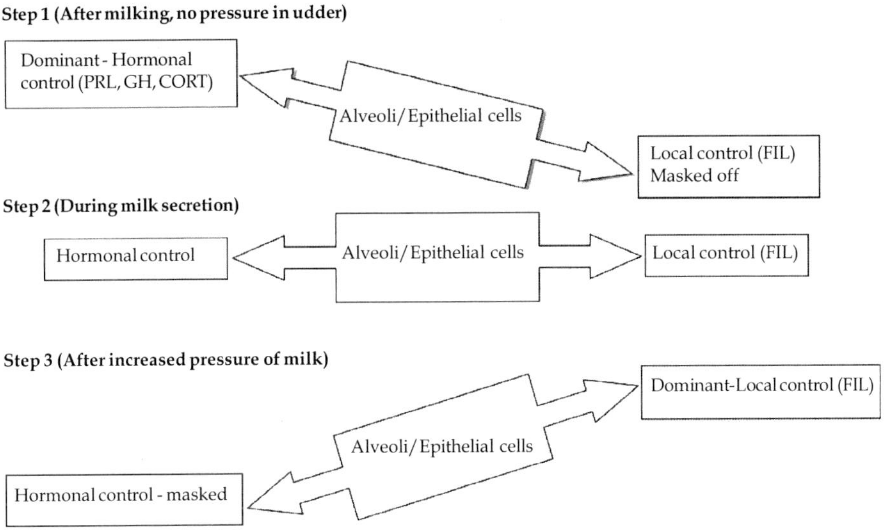

Figure. Mechanism of systermic and local factor (FIL) in milk secretion

Once milk is removed, the step 1, 2 and 3 are again repeated. FIL does not inhibit milk fat synthesis in-vivo but disrupts intracellurar protein trafficking thus reducing milk secretion. Milk accumulation reduces cell-surface receptors for prolactin and possibly IGF-I and alter sensitivity of the secretory cell to circulating lactogenic hormone complex. Prolactin and IGF-I are mammary mitogens, involved in the mammary cell survival through a complex interaction with the IGFBP5.

Serotonin

Serotonin (5-HT) is a hormone and neurotransmitter and is synthesized from L-tryptophan. It is a component of autocrine-paracrine homeostatic feedback mechanism which opposes hormonal stimulation of mammary gland development and milk secretion. Serotonin is a potent mammary vasoconstrictor and affects teat smooth muscle motility in bovines. Mammary epithelial cells with 5-HT reduce milk protein mRNA expression. The 5HT-1β, 2α, 2β, 4, and 7 receptors of serotonin in bovine mammary tissue have been reported. It is possible that some or all of these have direct or indirect effects on milk synthesis and secretion. 5-HT 7-receptor is present on the basolateral surface of human and mouse mammary epithelial cells and is involved in tight junction regulation.

❏❏❏

CHAPTER-14

Plasminogen activator-plasminogen-plasmin (PA-PG-PL) System

Milk production by the mammary gland depends on a complex interplay of lactogenic hormones and the stimulus induced by removal of milk from the udder by suckling or milking stimulus. Mothers regulate milk secretion in each mammary gland independently from the volume of milk suckled by the infant at each feed. Frequent milking of one udder half has no effect on milk secretion of the other half of udder in goats and cows suggesting that a local inhibitor in mammary gland controls milk secretion. Milk production also depends on external factors like emotional stress, heat stress, feed intake and water deprivation. In addition to FIL, milk secretion is regulated by plasminogen activator-plasminogen-plasmin (PA-PG-PL) system during summer stress in dairy animals.

The concentration of plasmin is high during late lactation, infrequent milking and interruption of milk removal. This pattern prompted researchers to investgate the role of plasmin in milk production. Plasmin exists in milk as a component of a complex system, including its zymogen *i.e.* plasminogen, plasminogen activators (PAs) and inhibitors of both plasmin and PAs. Plasmin originates from blood and enters milk in soluble form and then associates with the casein micelles because of its high affinity. Factors like lactation, seasonality, stress, diet and mastitis affect the plasmin concentration.

Regulation of milk secretion by plasmin

The involvement of plasminogen activator (PA)–plasminogen–plasmin system (PA-PG-PL) has been characterized in many biological fluids during the last decades in dairy cows. This system is intensively studied in the lysis of blood clots, regulation of cell activity and cell attachment in various tissues. Plasmin has trypsin-like activity and is mainly found in its inactive or zymogen form *i.e.* plasminogen. Plasmin concentration in fresh milk ranges from 0.1–0.7 mg/mL, while plasminogen to plasmin ratio in milk varies widely from 50:1 to 2:1. Plasmin is a major protease enzyme in milk and its concentration is high during late lactation. The conversion of plasminogen to plasmin is modulated by plasminiogen activator (PA), two types of which exist in mammals: urokinase type PA (u-PA) and tissue-type PA (t-PA). Plasmin, plasminogen, and t-PA are closely associated with the casein micelles whereas u-PA is associatedwith neutrophils. The inhibitors of PA and plasmin are in the milk serum known as plasminogen inhibitors. The close proximity of plasmin to its substrate ensures that hydrolysis is an efficient process and it is the primary agent of proteolysis in good quality milk. The association of t-PA with the casein micelle suggests a pivotal role of it in regulating plasmin activity under pathological conditions. However, u-PA activity increases during bacterial infection with increase in neutrophil numbers in the mammary gland. The optimum pH for plasmin is 7.5.

Plasminogen: Plasminogen is a single-chain glycoprotein with a molecular mass of 92 kDa. Plasminogen concentration in fresh milk varies from 0.8–2.8 mg/mL. Plasminogen is synthesized mainly in the liver and it circulates as inactive form in the vasculature. It is also found ubiquitously in other body fluids. Plasminogen thus secreted as a precursor, is cleaved by plasminogen activators at a single site to yield a two-chain plasmin held together by two disulfide bonds.

The main protein in milk is casein which is arranged as large colloidal particles commonly known as micelle. Four types of caseins (CN) are α-Casein, β-casein γ-casein and k-casein. β-CN is the preferred substrate for plasmin and its hydrolysis results in the production of γ-caseins and proteose–peptones. Milk has two third of β-casein and the rest is whey protein. Kappa-casein is resistant to proteolysis by plasmin. The insulin-like growth factor binding proteins (IGFBPs) interact with several proteins present in milk including β-casein, lactoferrin and transferrin. These interactions implicate the IGFBPs in the regulation of plasminogen activation since plasminogen and t-PA also bind to β-casein. An evidence exists regarding a close association between the PA–PG-PL system and gradual involution of mammary gland. The concentration of γ-caseins has been reported to be negatively correlated with milk yield in the declining phase of lactation, reflecting the gradual involution of the gland. β-CN f

(1–28) is negatively correlated with milk yield in the declining phase of lactation. It has been proposed that β–CNf (1–28) plays a role in the regulation of milk secretion. In bovines, the secretion of K^+, Na^+ and Cl^- determines approximately 40% of the driving force of water and the rest is determined by lactose. The lactose and monovalent ions are secreted into the lumen of the mammary gland mainly via vesicles. The apical membrane of epithelial cells contains K^+, Na^+ and Cl^- channels which are involved in the regulation of milk secretion. During heat stress, dehydration or emotional stress activates HPA causing the release of ACTH which releases cortisol from the adrenal gland. Cortisol stimulates the release of PA which converts plasminogen to plasmin. The plasmin induces formation of β-CN f (1–28) which is a potent blocker of K^+ channels in the apical membrane of mammary epithelial cells and decreases lactose synthesis. The production of β-CN f (1–28) by plasmin during the storage of milk in the udder represents between 8% and 12% of the total proteose–peptone fraction in whey and is resistant to further degradation by plasmin. The role of BCN fraction 1-28 has been experimently proved by infusion of a solution of casein digest enriched with β-CN f (1–28) into the cistern of cows, or infusion of pure β-CN f (1–28) into the cistern of goat, which resulted in a transient reduction in milk secretion after 8 hr. of infusion. The activation of hypothalamus–pituitary–adrenocortical axis by external stress liberates cortisol into the blood plasma, which induces the liberation of PA into the mammary cistern, where it activates the plasmin system and enhances the release of β-CN f (1–28) from β-CN. It is postulated that inhibition of K^+channels by β-CN f (1–28) triggers reduction in the secretion of lactose and monovalent ions into the lumen of the gland leading to decrease in milk volume. This rapid modulation of milk secretion increases the potential for survival in response to stress. The activation of plasmin (10–40% increase in activity) and the response induced by β-CN f (1–28) affects specifically fluid secretion (water, lactose and ions) only. It has no effect on lactose, fat and protein secretion, on the integrity of tight junctions and the leukocyte level of mammary gland. On the other hand, massive activation of plasmin activity (x150%) is associated with extensive degradation of casein, disruption of tight junctions, inflammatory responses (increasedleukocytes and NAGase activity) and a reduction in lactose concentration. The heat stress therefore increases plasmin, plasminogen activator concentration in milk and reduces the ratio of plasminogen to plasmin. Plasminogen activator concentration of milk is associated with the reduction in milk yield.

Its concentration is more during involution of mammary gland in cows. rBST treatment reduces production of PA.

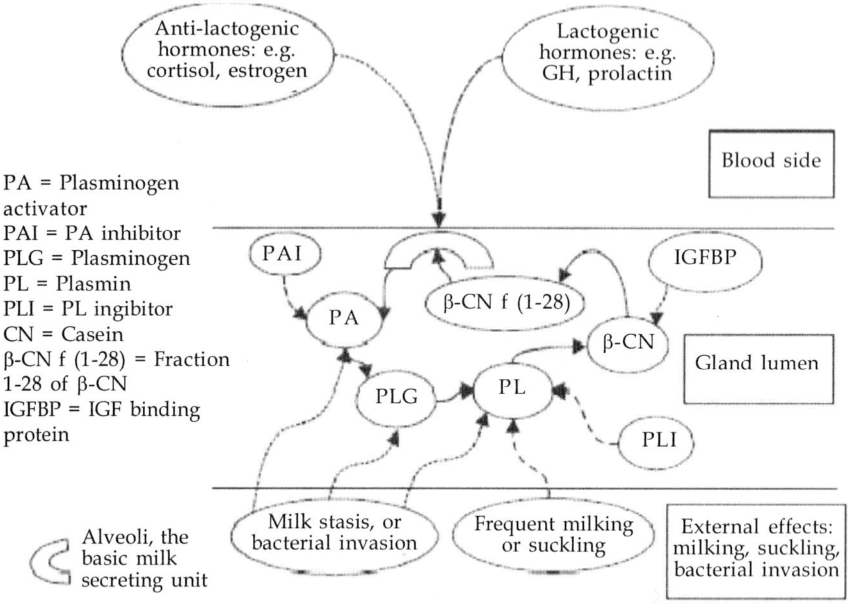

Overview of the PA-plasminogen-plasmin negative feedback mechanism that down-regulate milk secretion. Bold arrows indicate flow signal along the feedback loop, dotted arrows positive effects and dashed arrows suppressive effects).

Tight junctions

The tight junction (also called zonula occludens) is a 'gasket-like' structure. These junctions form the part of the complex and surround endothelial or epithelial cells. The junction forms a barrier that prevents vectorial movement of small molecules and ions between the basolateral and apical sides of cells when intact. The 'barrier'of tight junctions separate ions or small molecules differing in concentration on either side of the cell. These tight junctions also maintain polarised state of secretory cells, by preventing redistribution of plasma membrane components (e.g. ion channels and ion pumps) and maintain a difference in lipid and protein composition between the basal and apical side of the plasma membrane. The latter function of the tight junction is often referred to as its 'fence' function.

The junctions also prevent serum components from entering into milk and vice versa. Basal part of the cell has irregular feet which increase surface area of the epithelial cell and helps in increased up-take of nutrients from the ECF. The cells are attached closely to each other through tight junctions. The transport of the nutrients between the cells is negligible and nutrients are transported through the cell. Diseased condition *i.e.* mastitis or administration of oxytocin loosens the tight junctions and they become leaky to ions and lactose. During lactation, when the ducts and alveoli are filled with milk, the secretory epithelium is positioned between two very different environments: the milk, containing high concentration of lactose and low concentrations of sodium and chloride, and interstitial fluid containing low concentration of lactose and high concentrations of sodium and chloride. Thus, when tight junctions are disrupted the Na^+ concentration in the milk rises, whereas K^+ declines.

The tight junctions become 'leaky' during periparturient period and mammary gland involution. Further, tight junctions also leak after approximately 17 hr of milk accumulation in cows and 21 hr in goats. This increases in permeability leads to the reduction of milk secretion and protease enzyme activity in the milk increases. PPS activity increase by as much as 500% during the onset of involution, compared to 30% when cows were exposed to stress.

❑❑❑

Chapter-15

Involution of Mammary Gland

The involution of mammary gland occurs with the gradual loss of epithelial cell activity and its numer with advancement of lactation. This type of involution is refered as natural involution of mammary gland. It can be defined as acomplex multi-step process by which the mammary gland returns to its non-lactating state. Involution of mammary gland is characterized by two distinct physiological events.

i) Apoptosis of the secretory cells (programmed cell death)

ii) Proteolytic degradation of basement membrane of mammary gland

The involuton changes occur in a gradual manner with a loss of epithelial cells after peak lactation and decrease in suckling or milking. Involution can also be due to abrupt cessation of milking or sudden weaning. The involution involves morphological, ultrastructural and biochemical changes in the mammary gland after stoppage of milking. Mammary involution in the mouse is characterized by a rapid loss of tissue function and degeneration of the alveolar structure and loss of epithelial cells. The dead cells are rapidly cleared by phagocytes and mammary gland returns to its pre-pregnant state. Senile involution has been described in humans also. Physiology of the mammary glands during the dry period differs from that of lactation. The involution of mammary glands is classified into 3 phases:

- Active phase which occur after 24 h of cessation of milking in cow/ buffalo
- Steady phase – which occur after 3- 4 week of involution.
- Redevelopment and colostrogenesis phase – that begin -3 to -4 week prior to the parturition.

Active involution phase

The process of active involution begins with the stoppage of periodic milking during drying off in a lactating animal or weaning of young calves. Stoppage of milk removal results in milk stasis (accumulation of milk) leading to distension of the udder. This sets inflammatory changes, decreased synthesis of milk constituents, local chemical feedback by milk constituents, mechanical stress in udder and stretching of epithelial cells that lead to the loss of secretory activity. In cows, the active involution is completed by 21-30 days after drying off. During this phase milk continues to accumulate for a couple of days and volume of secretion in the gland increases for 2 to 4 days after drying-off, then declines rapidly over the next week.

Concentrations of milk-specific components- like lactose, caseins, α-lactalbumin, β-lactoglobulin and milk fat decline slowly during the first 2-3 wk of the dry period, but never disappear completely. Although lactose concentration declines more rapidly, the concentration of serum origin protein like immunoglobulins and serum albumin increases during the first week of involution. All classes of immunoglobulins (Ig) increase, including IgG1, IgG2, IgA, IgM. There is a transitory increase in the selective transport of IgG1 from about days 2 to 4 of involution. Increased serum albumin concentrations reflect increased permeability of tight junctions between epithelial cells. However, α-albumin concentration does not approach serum levels in milk indicating that permeability barriers are not completely destroyed.

NAGase (N-acetyl-β-D-glucosaminidase) activity increases during mammary involution. Its concentration can be used as an indicator of tissue changes during involution and inflammation, so it is considered as a parameter to monitor subclinical mastitis. NAGase, an intracellular lysosomal enzyme is secreted mainly by polymorphonuclear leukocytes, (neutrophils) during phagocytosis and by damaged epithelial cells during cell lysis. This enzyme is found in large quantities in the mammary gland during involution and inflammation.

Lactoferrin (LF) concentrations increase markedly during active involution. LF is an iron-binding protein which competes with bacteria for iron. This is the basis for lactoferrin's bacteriostatic action. Invading bacteria are forced to compete with LF for iron. For coliform bacteria, citrate: LF ratio is important. Citrate chelates with Fe so that bacteria can use the citrate-iron complex. During early involution citrate concentration declines, while LF concentration increases(citrate: LF ratio is low). LF may play a role in mammary gland by affecting phagocyte function. LF also limits the oxidative degeneration of cellular components that can occur during periods of tissue disruption such as during inflammation and involution.

Cells in secretion of a involuting mammary glands

Different types of cells migrate from blood into the mammry gland which acts as a scavenger for cell debris. Total leukocyte concentration in mammary secretion increases rapidly during early involution. Very few epithelial cells (<2%) are present in mammary secretions during involution, however most of the cells in the secretion are leukocytes.

Leukocytes in mammary glands

Polymorphonuclear neutrophils (PMN) are phagocytic in nature and predominate for the first 3-7 days of involution.

Macrophages are also phagocytes which predominate after 7 days of involution. They play a major role in removing large quantities of fat and cellular debris, including dead PMN. Macrophages are filled with ingested fat droplets during mammary involution and also present in colostrum at the time of parturition.

Lymphocytes are always present and their number increases parallel with the macrophages, which are the most predominant cell types during the mid-dry period. However, specific function of lymphocytes in involuting mammary glands is unknown.

Steady phase of involution

The length of steady state period (mid-dry period) depends upon the total length of the dry period in a cow or buffalo. Active involution takes about 4 weeks to complete followed by redevelopment stage that takes about 3 or 4 wk, then the dry period lasts 45-60 days. With 45-60 days dry period the steady state phase is very short or there is no steady state phase. When the mammary tissue undergoes active involution and the redevelopment phase begins simultaneously, then the dry period lasts less than 40 days.

Redevelopment and colostrogenesis

Redevelopment and colostrogenesis phase begins at about 3 to 5 weeks prepartum. It marks the transition from dry non-lactating state to the lactating state. The selective transport of IgG1 occurs through epithelial cells during the 2 weeks prepartum. Concentrations of milk protein, fat, citrate and lactose increase in second week prepartum, while a marked increase occurs 3 to 5 days before parturition. This phase is prone to intramammary infections again as mammary gland undergoes just opposite changes that occur during early involution stage. The fluid rich in protein and citrate accumulates in the udder during this phase. Lacteal secretion may leak from the teats if there is a bulk secretion. The removal of milk should not be done until calving. At this stage the mammary gland secretion have;

- Relatively few leukocytes
- Increased milk fat and casein concentrations
- High ratio of citrate : LF
- Low LF concentration
- Increased level of immunoglobulins with colostrum formation

Induced involution of mammary gland

When milking is abruptly stopped, the changes in the mammary gland are not normal and known as induced involution. Cessation of milk removal leads to increased pressure of milk which sets initiation of induced mammary involution process. An inflammatory change in mammary gland occurs due to acculation of milk and increased pressure. The intracellular accumulation of milk fat droplets and secretory vesicles takes place. Formations of large vacuoles occur in the epithelial cells within 48 hours of cessation of milking. The vacuoles persist for at least 14 days of involution and disappear by day 28 of active phase of involution. Macrophages mirgrate into the cell and leucocyte number increases. There is release of lysosomal enzymes causing the necrosis of cells. This results in the inhibition of milk secretion and a rapid decline in lactose concentration. It indicates the synthesis of lactose and the disruption of associated water transport mechanism soon after the cessation of milk removal. Total protein concentrations of milk increases in early involution because of water resorption and increased concentrations of lactoferrin, serum albumin and immunoglobulins. These proteins increase during involution in contrast to milk-specific proteins such as casein, whose synthesis is decreased. The luminal area of alveoli declines where as interalveolar stromal area increases due to absorption. Thus a substantial reduction in fluid volume in the gland occurs between days 3 -7 of involution. The cytoplasmic organelles involved in milk protein synthesis (Golgi apparatus) and secretion function (vesicles) also decrease but limited changes occur in organelles with metabolic function (ribosomes). This probably account for the reduction in luminal volume. By day 28 the collapsed alveolar structures have very small lumen in contrast to lactation. Histologically interalveolar connective tissue, fibroblasts and extra-cellular matrix increase and the intra-alveolar area decrease. General alveolar structure is maintained thoughout involution in the cow.

Table. Changes in Composition of Mammary Secretions during the Dry Period

Milk component	Active Involution	Steady State Involution	Redevelopment and Colostrogenesis
Lactose	decreasing	low	increasing (late)
Milk Proteins	decreasing	low	increasing
Milk Fat	decreasing	low	increasing
Udder fluid volume	decreasing	low	increasing
Concentrations of:			
Milk components	decreasing	low	increasing
Leukocytes	increasing	high	low
Lactoferrin	increasing	high	low
Immunoglobulins	increasing	high	increasing

Myoepithelial cells (MEC) survive during involution as cells are resistant to involution. Mammary gland epithelium is composed of an inner layer of secretory cells (luminal) and an outer layer of myoepithelial cells (MEC) bordering the basal lamina which separates the epithelial layer from the extracellular matrix. MECs have cytokeratin filaments akin to smooth muscle cells. MECs are involved in mammary gland morphogenesis in all developmental stages, modulating proliferation and differentiation of luminal cells. They limit cancer growth, invasiveness and neoangiogenesis. MEC takes part in the formation of extracellular matrix, certain proteinases and their inhibitors. MECs are regarded as natural cancer suppressors through maspin protein and stabilize normal structure of the mammary gland.

❑❑❑

Chapter-16

Apoptosis

Apoptosis the programmed cell death (PCD) is a physiological cell loss process during mammary gland involution. It is achieved after the natural weaning/litter removal in rodents, after weaning in sow and during drying off in goat and cow. Apoptosis is both a natural and systematic method of cell suicide which takes place during normal morphogenesis, tissue remodelling and in response to infection or irreparable cell. Two distinct types of cell death- apoptosis and necrosis occur, which can be distinguished by morphological, biochemical and molecular changes in dying cells. Apoptosis is characterized by morphological changes like nuclear and cytoplasmic condensation, nuclear fragmentation, formation of apoptotic bodies and cleavage of chromatin into discrete sized oligonucleosome fragments by a calcium dependent endonuclease and appearance of oligonucleosomal DNA laddering in ethidium bromide stained gels. DNA laddering characteristic of apoptosis has been detected in goat mammary tissue during early and late lactation while it occurs in cows during late lactation. Recent advances in lactation reveal that the cause of declining epithelial cell number is due to the imbalance between cell proliferation and cell removal. The persistency of lactation and the rate of decline in milk yield with advancing lactation is influenced by the rate of apoptosis in the lactating gland. Removal of secretory epithelial cells by apoptosis is a normal physiological event in the ruminant mammary gland during lactation. However, factors that determine the rate of cell death by apoptosis are not characterized completely. Factors like frequency of milking, oxidative stress and nutrition, influence the cell survival after peak lactation. Reproductive hormones viz. oestradiol and progesterone maintain the mammary ductal and alveolar integrity during the dry period but allow apoptosis and cell replacement. In the adult mammary gland, p63 is highly expressed in the basal cell layer that comprises myoepithelial and interspersed stem/progenitor cells. p63 is a prosurvival factor in the adult mammary gland during post-lactational involution, affecting PI-MECs.

The p63 is essential in vivo for the survival and maintenance of parity-identified mammary epithelial cells (PI-MECs), a pregnancy-induced heterogeneous population that survives post-lactation involution. P63 contain multipotent progenitors that give rise to alveoli and ducts in subsequent pregnancies. PI-MECs are an interesting cellular subset because they survive involution.After involution, PI-MECs are present exclusively in the luminal layer of mammary ducts. During pregnancy, PI-MECs contribute to the luminal layer but not the basal layer of alveolar lobules. However, more reseach needs to be carried out on PI-MECs to relate it with persistency of lactation in different species.

The process of involution involve initiation of extensive cell death to remove the milk-producing epithelial cells of udder (1st phase) and this is followed by 2nd phase in which influx of macrophages and immune cells breakdown extracellular matrix and remodelling of blood vessels takes place. The other changes includes replenishment of adipocyte of mammary gland fat pad an removal of residual milk, and cell debris by phagocytises. There is proteolytic degradation of basement membrane of the mammary gland. It has been found that apoptosis remain almost absent during lactation but apoptotic cell appears on day 2 of involution and remain at least functional upto day 8 of involution. During this period the β-casein gene expression decline. In mice, the expression of sulphated glycoprotein-2 (SGP-2), interleukin-1β converting enzyme and tissue inhibitor of metallo-proteinases-1 is up-regulated on day 2. It has been shown that administration of glucocorticoid (hydrocortisone) inhibits mammary gland involution by inhibiting the wave of apoptotic cells in lumina of mammary gland and apoptosis-associated genes *SGP-2* and *ICE. However,* matrix metalloproteinases (MMPs) stromelysin-1, stromelysin-3, gelatinase A and serine proteinase urokinase-type plasminogen activator (uPA) increase during involution.

❑❑❑

Chapter-17

Plasma Energy Metabolites During Lactation

Lactation is a physiological state associated with significant metabolic adaptations and changes in energy balance. A major increase in energy demand, along with a decrease in adaptive thermogenesis, occurs during lactation. The adaptation has been considered as an energy-sparing mechanism to facilitate the availability of energy for milk production.

Plasma NEFA and glucose are important energy markers for a dairy animal. Factors like infections, stress, or trauma increase NEFA concentration and fat in liver. As the concentration of NEFA in blood increases around calving or in early lactation, more NEFA are oxidized to carbon dioxide to provide energy for the liver or is partially oxidized to produce ketone bodies that serve as fuels for other tissues. Alternatively it can be reconverted to storage fat as triglycerides. NEFA concentrations begin to rise 7 days before calving, reaching peak levels after 3 to 4 days of calving and decline to lower levels by 14 to 21 days postpartum. The normal values of NEFA for cows in positive energy balance are less than 200 μM. NEFA values increases to 200 to 300 μM before a week of calving and peak at 800 to 1200 μM per litre on the day of calving due to hormonal changes and the stress of parturition. NEFA values of greater than 700 μM beyond 7 days postcalving indicate severe NEBAL or health problems and are an indicative of transition. NEFA values should be below 300 μM three weeks after calving. A high ratio of GH: insulin in early lactation of cow induces mobilization of fatty acids from adipose tissue. Adipose tissue is highly sensitivite to lipolytic signals of catecholamines in early lactation. The percentage of blood NEFA utilized by the liver is fairly constant, hence the concentration of NEFA in blood reflects the degree of adipose tissue mobilization.

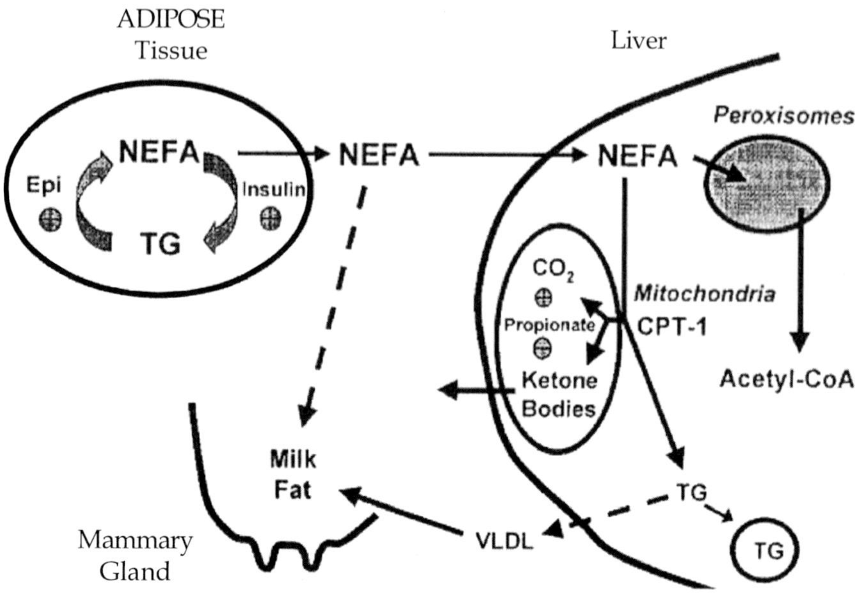

Plus signs (+) = stimulatory effects (-) signs = inhibitory effects

Plasma glucose

Glucose availability is a precondition for high milk production. The forage-fed ruminants absorb very little glucose from their feed in contrast to nonruminants. Glucose requirements of ruminants are mainly met through glucose synthesis, which predominantly occurs in the liver utilizing its precursors absorbed after fermentation and digestion of the diet. Therefore, glucose metabolism represents a balance between glucose requirement for milk production and glucose carbon supply from the diet, which is integrated by the liver. There is a considerable capacity for starch digestion in the small intestine and subsequent increases in glucose supply to the cow. But the increased glucose supply is used to support body fat and protein retention and not for greater milk production. This response is accompanied by changes in insulin concentration and may have important implications for the metabolic health and reproductive success of the early lactating cow. The contribution of propionate dominates among the glucose precursors. In transition dairy cows, the contributions of lactate, alanine and glycerol to liver glucose synthesis were greatest at 11 days postpartum; reflecting negative body energy balance, but the required contribution of other amino acids to glucose synthesis during early lactation is minimum. Milk yield and metabolic heat production decrease under high ambient temperatures in cows. The reduction in metabolism is associated with a decrease in voluntary feed intake and adaptation of endocrine mechanisms. Thyroxine, growth hormone, triiodothyronine and glucocorticoids decrease in cattle exposed to heat stress. Plasma insulin concentrations are lower in nonlactating cows, unaffected in heifers and higher in nonlactating sheep following exposure to a hot environment. In lactating cows, plasma insulin concentration does not correlate with the utilization of glucose by the mammary gland and the whole body utilization of glucose mostly occurs through non-insulin-dependent pathways.

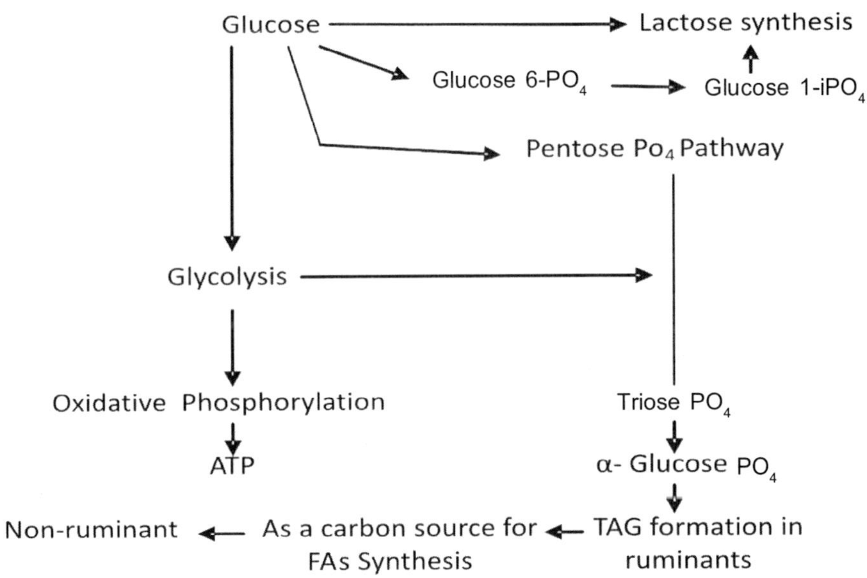

Figure. Glucose Metabolic Pathway in epithelial cell of a mammary gland

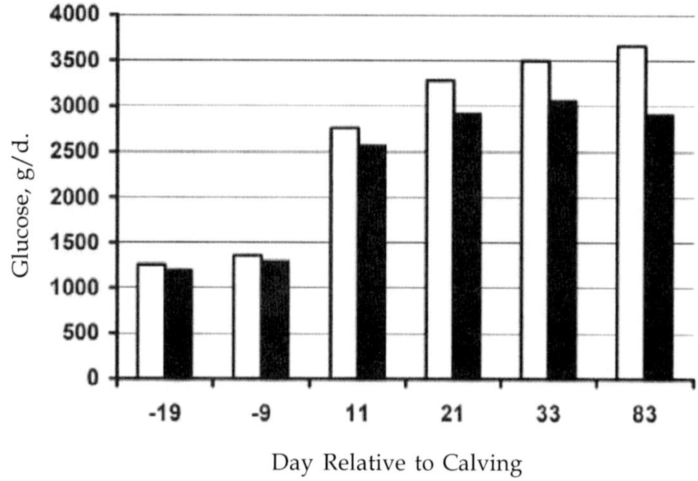

Figure. Liver glucose release (open bars) and estimated glucose requirement (solid bars) in transition dairy cows (Reynolds et al., 2003)

Insulin secretion is inhibited during lactation. Moreover, insulin and glucagon secretion of dairy cattle has also been reported to differ depending on the physiological state under normal ambient temperatures. Insulin secretion and action probably change with the decrease in milk production following exposure of dairy cows to hot environments. The concentrations of insulin and glucagon in venous blood are the result of the rate of release from the pancreas and the rate of removal by the remainder of the body, especially the liver. Experimental evidences indicate that early lactation dairy cow has a greater capacity for glucose metabolism than is provided by voluntary feed intake of average diets, but all available glucose is not partitioned to the mammary gland.

❑❑❑

Chapter-18

Oxytocin

Oxytocin is a short polypeptide hormone, $C_{43}H_{66}N_{12}O_{12}S_2$ released from the posterior lobe of the pituitary gland that stimulates the contraction of smooth muscles of the uterus during labor and facilitates ejection of milk from the mammary glands during nursing. It is a peptide hormone of nine amino acids with a sequence of cysteine - tyrosine - isoleucine - glutamine - asparagine - cysteine - proline - leucine - glycine. The cysteine residues form a sulfur bridge. Oxytocin has a molecular mass of 1007 daltons. One international unit (IU) of oxytocin is equivalent to about 2 micrograms of pure peptide. The structure of oxytocin is very similar to that of vasopressin (cysteine - tyrosine - phenylalanine - glutamine - asparagine - cysteine - proline - arginine - glycine), also a nonapeptide with a sulfur bridge, however, vasopressin sequence differ from oxytocin by 2 amino acids.

Oxytocin is the first naturally-occurring peptide hormone to be synthesized, a feat for which Du Vigneaud received Nobel Prize in 1955. Oxytocin is synthesized mainly in specialized magnocellular neurons in the supraoptic and paraventricular nucleus of hypothalamus, separate from the vasopressin-synthesizing neurons. Both oxytocin and ADH are packaged into granules and secreted along with carrier proteins called neurophysins from the posterior pituitary gland. It is also secreted within the brain and from a few other tissues, including ovaries and testes.

Oxytocin receptors

The Oxytocin receptor (OXTR) functions as an inducer of uterine contractions and milk ejection. OXTR is expressed by the myoepithelial cells of mammary glands. It is also expressed in myometrium and endometrium of uterus at the end of pregnancy. In some mammals, oxytocin receptors are found in the kidney and heart. In humans, the oxytocin receptor is encoded by the OXTR gene. Oxytocin receptor is also widespread throughout the central nervous system and modulates a variety of behaviors. These include responses to stress and anxiety, social memory and recognition, sexual and aggressive behaviors, bonding (affiliation) and maternal behavior. Oxytocin agonists are demoxytocin and carbetocin peptides. Oxytocin appears to stimulate the growth of myoepthelial cells both *in vitro* and *in vivo*.

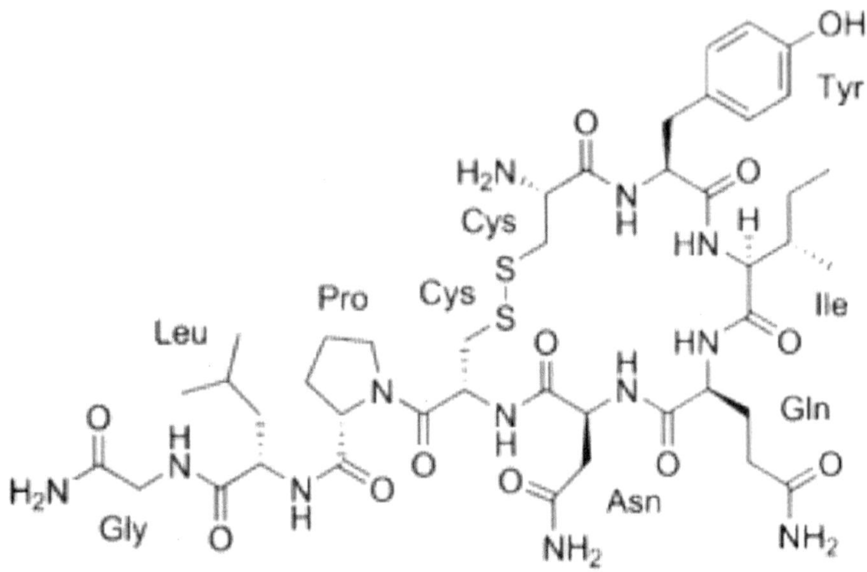

Figure. Structure of oxytocin

Physiological functions of oxytocin

Oxytocin has been studied more in females and mediates three major effects:

A. Milk ejection

Milk is initially secreted into small sacs within the mammary gland called alveoli, from which it must be ejected for consumption or harvesting. Mammary alveoli are surrounded by smooth muscle (myoepithelial) cells which have oxytocin receptors. Oxytocin stimulates contraction of myoepithelial cells causing milk to be ejected into the ducts and cisterns.

In the bovine mammary gland about 80% of milk is stored in the alveoli (alveolar milk) and is transferred into milk cistern only by neuroendocrine reflex. Oxytocin is released from the pituitary gland in response to tactile teat/milking stimulus. The amount of milk left in the udder (residual milk) can be removed only by exogenous i.v. administration of oxytocin at supra-physiological dosage. In cows or buffaloes natural oxytocin release/minute is 15 to 90 pg/mL which persists only for a few minutes.

B. Uterine smooth muscle contraction at birth

At the end of gestation, the uterus must contract vigorously for a prolonged period of time in order to deliver the fetus. During the later stages of gestation, there is an increase in abundance of oxytocin receptors on uterine smooth muscle cells, which is associated with increased "irritability" of the uterus. Oxytocin is released during labor when fetus stimulates the cervix and vagina. It enhances contraction of uterine smooth muscle to facilitate parturition or birth of calf. In cases where uterine contractions are not sufficient to complete delivery, physicians and veterinarians administer oxytocin (pitocin) to stimulate uterine contractions. However, a great care must be exercised in such situations to ensure that the fetus can indeed be delivered and to avoid rupture of uterus.

C. Maternal behavior

Oxytocin play important role in establishing the affinity bond between mothers and offspring immediately after birth. It is also important that non-lactating females do not manifest such nurturing behavior. The same events that affect the uterus and mammary gland at the time of birth also affect the brain. The oxytocin level and its action within the brain plays a major role in establishing maternal behavior. During parturition, there is an increase in concentration of oxytocin in cerebrospinal fluid.

Neuroendorcrine reflex

The neuroendorcrine reflex release oxytocin hormone and involve two components i.e. i) nervous system and ii) endocrine system pathways. The nervous pathway involve transmission of sensory stimuli of suckling or hand milking within a few milliseconds to the hypothalamus (brain) via a spinal reflex arc and then to the posterior pituitary gland leading to the release of oxytocin into (Figure). The oxytocin is synthesized in the supraoptic and paraventricular hypothalamic nuclei and is stored in the terminal nerve endings of the neurons which lie in the posterior pituitary gland. The blood oxytocin reaches the udder and binds with the OXTR on myoepitheal cells and contract myoepithelial cells. Contraction of myoepithelial cells lead to collapse of alveoli and squeezing of milk into small ducts. These ducts shorten and widen and the milk rushes into the gland cistern. Only alveolar and small ductal milk is expelled by the action of oxytocin on the myoepithelium. There is no contraction of large ducts or cisterns. The milk stored in lumen of alveoli passes into the larger ducts and gland cistern and causes engorgement of udder. Milk ejection process is therefore important in dairy cows because about 80% of the milk is available only after ejection. The washing of teats and lower udder prior to milking also causes release of oxytocin and aid to milk ejection.

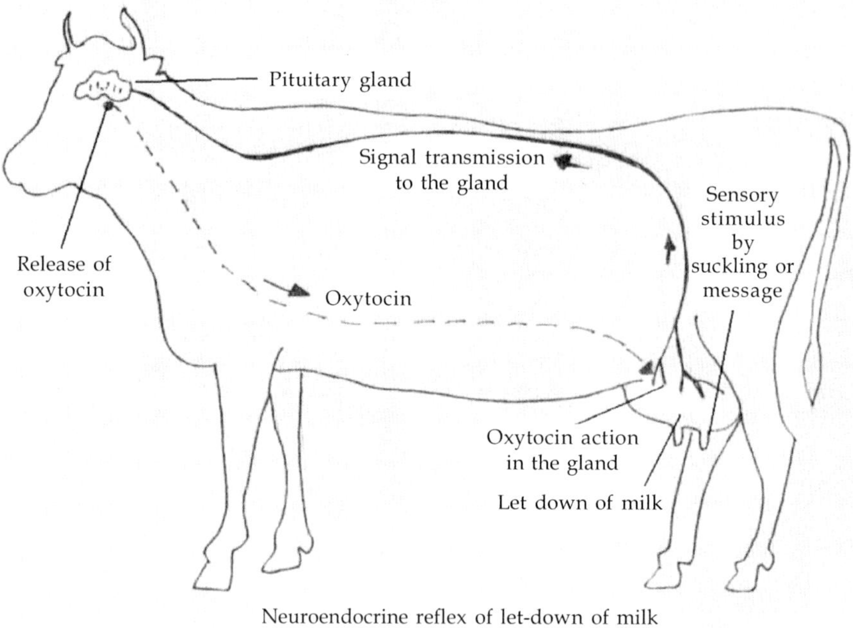

Neuroendocrine reflex of let-down of milk

Inhibition of oxytoxcin release

Factors like acute stress/parturition stress, extreme cold, hot-temperature; improper handling of animal at milking, sound of firecrackers and abnormal sounds can inhibit oxytocin release. Psychological stress or pain also decreases milk output. In humans, ethyl alcohol is a potent inhibitor of oxytocin release. Morphine also inhibits let-down reflex. Stress or disturbed milking operations release adrenal catecholamine's (epinephrine or nor-epinephrine) which reaches to mammary gland and causes i) increased tone in mammary ducts ii) vasoconstriction of blood vessels. Both the effects result in less blood supply in mammary gland. In addition epinephrine binds with the receptors of oxytocin located on myoepithelium cells. This leaves fewer receptor sites for binding of oxytocin hormone. Due to these reasons oxytocin effect on myoepithelium cells is effectively blocked. This is called *peripheral inhibition* of let down of milk. This type of inhibition cannot be corrected by administration of exogenous oxytocin in cows and buffaloes. The second type of inhibition is known as *central inhibition of let down of milk* in which release of oxytocin from the hypothalamic nuclei is impaired. Such inhibition can be corrected by exogenous oxytocin.

The myoepithelial cells have oxytocin receptors binding site and assists in expulsion of milk from the udder. These myoepithelial cells have no nerve connection. They are arranged in two ways.

i) In a starlike (stellate) fashion around the alveoli to achieve maximum squeezing action to collapse it which is called implosion.
ii) In a longitudinal arrangement along the small ducts to effect a shortening and widening of these small tubes. This aids in the expulsion of the milk from the collapsed alveolus by increasing the size of the passage. In contrast to the myoepithelial cells within the udder, smooth muscle are found around blood vessels, small and large ducts and sinuses.

Factors affecting release of oxytocin

Milk ejection reflex is also pre-programmed or conditioned by the brain. The rattling of milk buckets, washing of udders, feeding of concentrate, sight and approach of milker, message of teat, application of milking machine, time of milking, place of milking, entry of cows in milking byre lead to conditioned reflex/stimuli meaning that milking is about to commence. Accordingly when brain receives correct message, it automatically triggers release of oxytocin. Any stress or disturbance leads to impairement in letdown of milk. Buffaloes are very sensitive to the surroundings of the milking enviornemnt. This may lead to impairment in let-down of milk and less milk yields. Milk let-down reflex of dairy animals is very easily retarded by any external stimuli which disrupt the normal milking operations. It is often said that a buffalo or cow "holds up" her milk. This is not possible since the cow has no voluntary control over the let-down process. But disturbed milking operations, unfamiliar surroundings, rough handling of animal, loud and unfamiliar noise, pain, discomfort and irritation can decrease or terminate let-down of milk by the mechsnim which is being mentioned above. Cows and buffaloes handled gently and milked carefully at regular intervals normally do not suffer from milk ejection problem.

An effective milk ejection reflex is essential to achieve fast and efficient milking. Milk ejection reflex usually takes place in 20 to 40 seconds after the initial stimulation (udder wiping) and lasts for about 6 minutes. It is most important that the milk is removed within this time while this reflex is operating. There is a 30 to 60 seconds lag period between applying the machine and contraction of the alveoli. However, passive withdrawal of milk occurs during this interval. This kind of lag may be particularly beneficial when milking high-producing cows since the reduction of pressure within the cisterns ensure milk flow from the alveoli. Once the effect of oxytocin wears off, milk that has not been removed flow back from the sinuses of udder into the ducts and eventually into the alveoli. The amount of milk left in udder after normal milking is called residual milk and it can be removed only after oxytocin administration. The residual milk is rich in fat contents and its amount vary in different breeds.

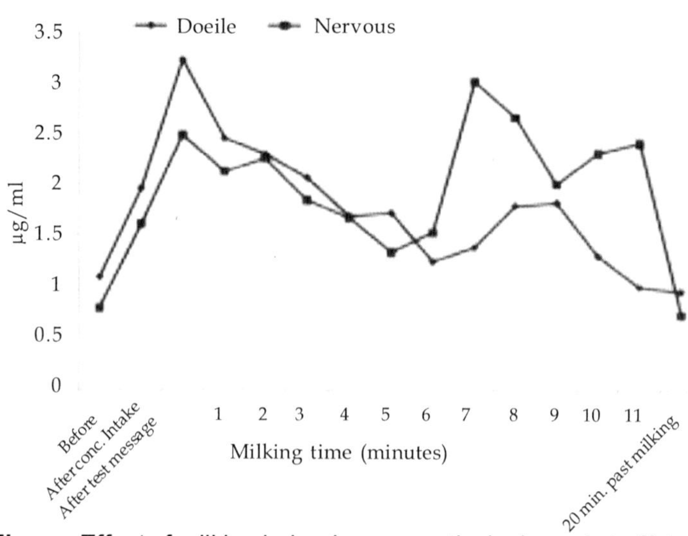

Figure. Effect of milking behaviour on cortisol release in buffaloes

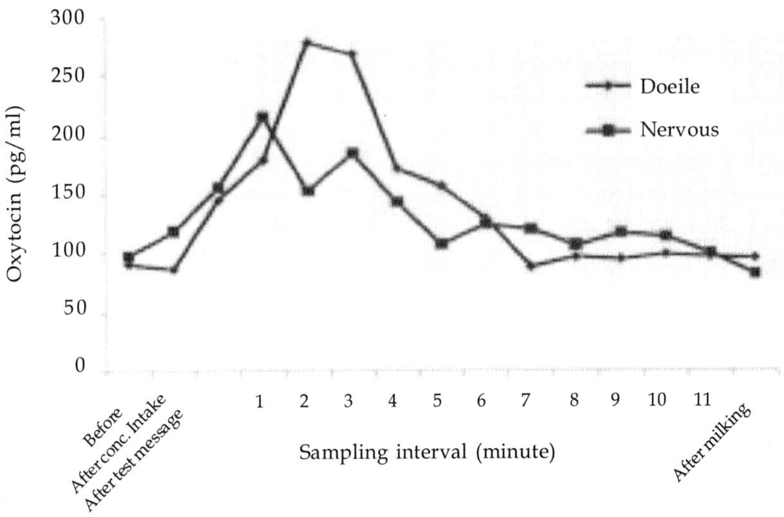

Figure. Effect of milking behaviour on plasma oxytocin release in Murrah buffaloes

Role of milk removal

Milk synthesis and milk removal are closely associated. If milking of a cows or buffalo is not done at regular intervals, the milk yield decline due to accumulation of milk in the udder. Contrary to this regular milking operation ensures full removal of milk and more release of hormones at milking. Thus a vital part in maintenance of lactation is removal of milk at regular intervals. Milk removal is associated with the passive withdrawal of milk from the alveoli into gland and teat cisterns and ducts of udder. The ejection of milk from the alveolar lumen is being achieved by teat message or udder message.

Passive withdrawal

In this phase of milking the active co-operation of the cow is not required. Cow's nose and eyes transmit signals to the brain by nerves. This causes the brain to release oxytocin into the bloodstream. Nerve endings in the skin of the udder and teats are stimulated by washing/ wiping of udder, the slipping-on of the teats cups and by pressure of the teat liner on the walls of the teat. The teat sphincter at the tip of the teat then opens and milk begins to pass out into the milk tube. This phase, which is activated by the nerves, begins about 5 to 10 seconds after the udder and teats have been stimulated. The nervous reflex brings about a squeezing of the ducts by the smooth muscle and the milk within the ducts is pushed into the udder cisterns. Since dairy cow has a relatively large cistern, 40 to 50% of the total milk yield may be obtained during this passive withdrawal phase.

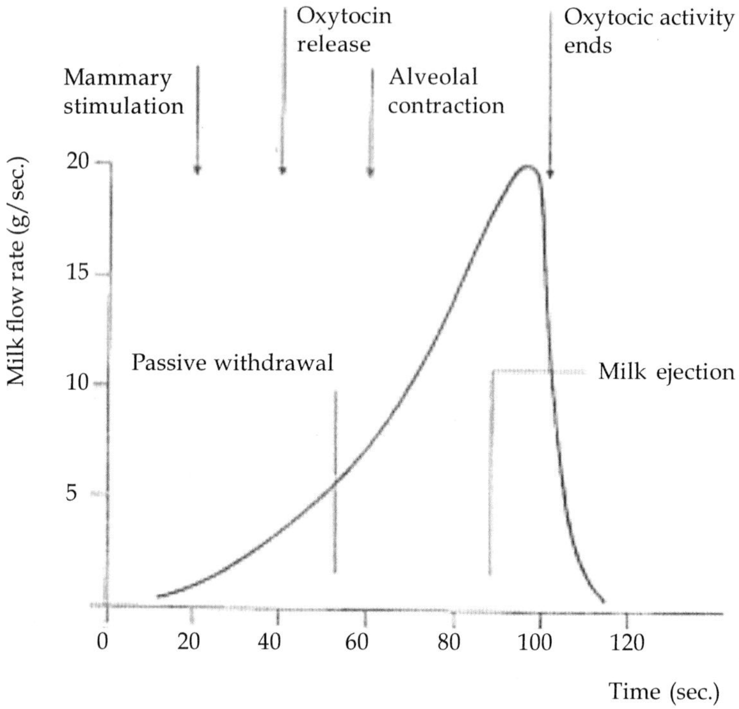

Pattern of milk flow from the udder (Whittemore, 1980)

Oxytocin concentration

The stimulus from the milking machine results in an adequate release of oxytocin for maximum milk ejection and a normal milk yield. The oxytocin concentration in the blood plasma declined rapidly after peak concentration. Oxtyocin concentration is maximum within 2-3 minutes of tactile stimuli and therefore hand milking or teat cup should be applied immediately. Oxytocin reach peak level within 2-3 minutes of milking and decrease to below 2.5 μU/ml by 5 minutes after teat cup application and toless than 0.01 μU/ml 5 minutes post milking. Reports indicate that peak oxytocin concentration decrease with advancing lactation non- significantly in HF dairy cows. During pregnancy the maternal oxytocin level (29.1 ± 2.6 pg/ml) are significantly lower than fetal oxytocin levels (45.8 ± 4.3 pg/ml). The concentration of milk oxytocin in dairy cows administered oxytocin (25 or 50 IU) prior to milking are very low and below the assay detection limit. Milk could be considered safe for human consumption although in one study OT was found to be quite stable at pasteurization temperatures in OT spiked milk of dairy cows. A significant correlation (r = 0.2523, p <0.05) between paired maternal oxytocin and fetal oxytocin levels throughout late pregnancy have been reported.

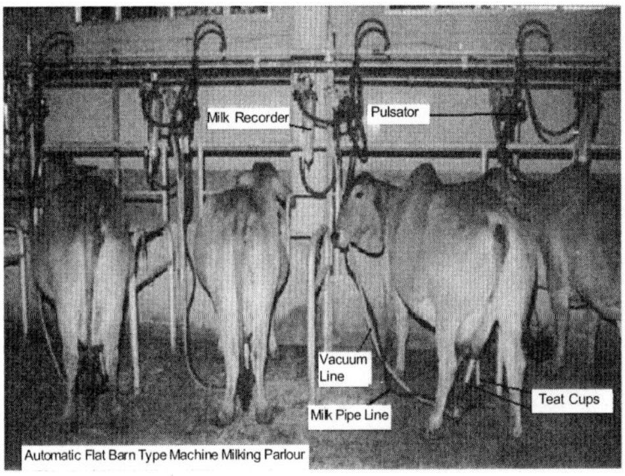

Sahiwal milking cows in a Flat Barn Milking Parlour System

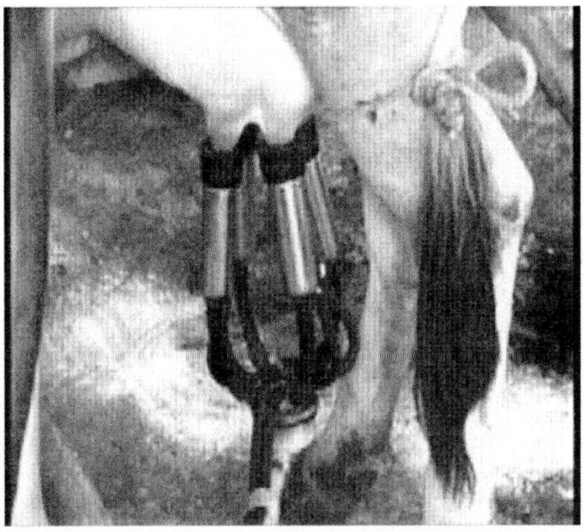

Teat cups attached to teats

Milking temperament

Buffaloes are different form cattle in milking characteristics and behavior at milkig. Murrah buffaloes have smaller cisternal area sizes and cisternal fraction of milk than cattle. Teats of buffaloes are longer and thicker and have longer teat canals. Before commencement of milking operations the teats of buffaloes are flaccid and empty due to the small cisternal fraction of milk, while during milk ejection remarkable increase in teat dimensions and cisternal cavity area occurs. Milk flow in buffaloes commences only after the alveolar fraction of milk is emptied. Due to this reason the buffaloes require more teat message to let-down alveolar milk. Milking also results in more pronounced release of oxytocin, prolactin and cortisol which is similar to reports in cattle. Attaching the milking cluster prior to milk ejection could lead to higher teat penetration in teats without milk. To prevent irritation to the teat tissue due to machine milking without milk flow at high vacuum levels, the milk removal has to be synchronised with milk ejection. Buffaloes respond well to mechanisation of daily management activities and could perform well if their species-specific requirements are fulfilled.

Half life of oxytocin

The oxytocin concentration is essential for letdown of milk but is very low in blood of lactating animals. Milking or suckling stimulus causes a marked increase in the blood oxytocin concentrations in mammals. But oxytocin in the blood stream disappears quite rapidly. This is brought about either by destruction of the hormone in the body or by elimination from the blood. The kidneys, liver and mammary gland are mainly involved in removing the oxytocin from the bloodstream through oxytocinase. Oxytocin disappears rapidly from the circulation thus posing problems for its accurate estimation. In cows half life of oxytocin ranges from 0.8 to 1.30 minutes and in humans the value is about 5 minutes. The half-life in the circulation for intravenously injected hormone is 40 sec. to 4 min. in a variety of species. The concentration of oxytocin in the blood is dependent on the time interval after release from hypothalamus. It reaches peak concentration in the blood approximately one minute after stimulation of animal and the concentrations are generally undetectable after five minutes of milking.

Residual milk

Residual milk is high in fat content because when the milk is stored in the gland then insoluble and light weight contents of milk such as fat, fat soluble vitamins etc. come on upper side and the milk from lower side is removed first thus the upper milk is left as residual milk and is high in fat content. First drawn milk may have only 1-2 % fat, whereas, at the end, fat percentage between 5-10 % is common. Residual milk may have as high as 20 %. Amount of residual milk varies from breed to breed. Buffaloes have 0.4 to 7 % residual milk while cattle and crossbred cows have 5-15 % residual milk. Older cows have higher percentage of residual milk than first calf heifers. The percentage of residual milk is also higher in low producer than in high producers. For dairying purposes animals are preferred having low retention or low percentage of residual milk. Time delays between udder preparation and milking results in higher residual milk, lower peak flow rates and low milk and fat yields. The removal of residual milk itself has a profound effect on the subsequent secretion rate, and the concentration of butterfat. In addition to economic loss, milk remaining in the mammary gland may harbor micro-organisms and leads to more SCC and increased incidence of mastitis.

Milk has two phases-aqueous and the lipid phase. Compared to the aqueous phase of milk, milk lipid has a lower specific gravity, thus milk lipid rises in the upper part of milk phases. The phase difference in milk accounts in part for the variation in fat content as it leaves the udder. Fat droplets pass less readily from the udder than the aqueous phase and accumulate in the gland cistern to upper ducts and in the alveoli. As a general rule the residual milk is a percentage of milk and its incidence is affected by completeness of milk ejection, resulting variations even within individual. Thus diurnal variation in fat concentration of milk at AM and PM milking is as a result of carry over effects of residual milk. The greater the cow's production, the wider is the variation in fat percentage found in first and last drawn milk. Milk drawn with the shortest previous milking interval will have the highest fat content because the high fat milk remaining from the previous milking is diluted less by the milk produced in the shorter milking interval. The variation in fat percentage from one milking to another milking for a cow is probably the best indicator of completeness of milk ejection and removal of available milk. Reduction in residual milk results in higher daily yield except in the first part of lactation, when only a higher fat content in milk could be demonstrated.

Effect of exogenous oxytocin on milk production

Use of oxytocin for milking has been found to disrupt the integrity of mammary gland epithelium. Certain substances like sodium, chloride, bicarbonate pass into milk, whereas substances like potassium and lactose being higher in milk passes into blood. Further oxytocin bind with greater affinity (8-10 fold) with myo-epithelial cells of mammary gland and have ability to respond to oxytocin by shortening of elongated surface projections. The effect of oxytocin on milk production varies considerably. Few reports indicate increase in milk yield and decrease in fat content of milk after injection of oxytocin, whereas SNF and lactose percentage decrease. But method of oxytocin administration had no effect on the yields of residual milk or on its chemical composition in crossbred cows and buffaloes. Oxytocin in lower doses (1 I.U.) may not have any ill effect on the health of dairy animals due to very short half life. Use of exogenous oxytocin may affect the length of estrus cycle. The intramuscular administration of oxytocin does not affect feed and water intake, milk production and composition of buffaloes and cattle when used in small doses (1-5

IU/d). Frequent use of oxytocin for milking in few parts of the country may also lead to productive problems (Table). This matter is debatable but needs immediate attention of the animal scientists. The farmers have misapprehension that use of oxytocin increases milk production of cows and buffaloes. Rather use of oxytocin decrease milk yield, milk fat percentage and the animals may suffer with mastitis incidence.

Table. Reasons to use oxytocin by the owner of the animal

Reason	Buffalo (N-60)	Cattle (N-60)
Increase Milk yield	(25) 41.66%	(20) 33.33%
Dead Fetus	(2) 3.33%	(6) 10%
Difficult Birth	(13) 21.66%	(18) 30%
Retention of Placenta	(11) 18.33%	(9) 15%
Milk let down	(9) 15%	(7) 11.66%

Table. Effect of oxytocin on milk yield and fat percentage in buffalo and cattle

	Ist day	1 week	1 month	3 month	6 month	9 month	1 year
Milk yield, L	12 (9-18)	12.3 (10-23)	10 (10-21)	9.3 (10-20.5)	9 (8-17)	8.6 (6-14)	8 (3-10)
Milk fat, %	8.5%	8%	8%	7%	5.7%	5%	4.2%
Mastitis	(23) 38.33%	(11) 18.33%	(19) 31.66%	(21) 35%	(16) 26.66%	(12) 20%	(18) 30%
Milk yield, L	18 (9-21)	18 (11-21)	16.8 (8-20)	16 (12-22)	15.4 (10-18)	13.9 (8-17)	11 (6-10)
Milk fat %	6.2%	6.2%	5.8%	5.5%	4.9%	4%	3.7%
Mastitis	(12) 20%	(21) 35%	(14) 23.33%	(16) 26.66%	(9) 15%	(4) 6.66%	(7) 11.66%

Cattle (n = 60); Buffalo n = 60

(Mustafa *et al.*, 2008).

It has been reported that frequent use of oxytocin results in various reproductive disorders in buffalo and cattle viz., follicular ovarian cyst 18.33%, carpus Luteum cyst 28.33%, retention of placenta 11.66%, anestrous 16.66% and repeated estrus 25% in buffalo and follicular cyst 26.66%, corpus luteum cyst 23.33%, retention of placenta 8.33%, anestrous 18.33% and repeated estrus 23.33%, respectively.

❑❑❑

Chapter-19

Hippocampus Neuroprotection During Lactation

Lactation is associated with increased levels of oxytocin, prolactin, progesterone and glucocorticoids. During pregnancy and lactation, the fluctuation of the ovarian hormonal levels is modified while circadian secretion of corticoids is lost. Neuroprotection in the hippocampus during lactation might involve actions of any one or a combination of these hormones on the maternal brain. Maternal brain adjusts through neruoendocrine, automatic and behavour responses and neuroplasticity for the neuroprotection. Plasticity is defined as the intrinsic property of nervous system which involves systematic functional and morphological changes in the brain in response to afferent inputs. The hippocampus undergoes remodeling of cell structure in hypothalamic nuclei and limbic structure associated with lactation. In limbic system more expression of materinal behavour and more stress response occur in terms of neurotransmission, stress response, anxiety, cognitive performances and the learning and memory process of it takes place. The dorsal part of hippocampus of maternal brain is more affected due to more Kainic acid (KA) during pregnancy. Expression of KA and glutamate and their binding to receptors decline during preganancy. KA an agonist to glutamate depolarizes pre and post synaptic neurons through glutamate. It induces excitotoxic cell damage in hippocampus; disrupt mitochondria function and induce apoptosis of cell. The cell death is induced through necrotic and apoptotic patheway. The animal adaptive behavour response also alters to satisfy the demand of litter/calf. The CA1, CA3 and CA4 part of hippocampus are more sensitive to KA toxic effect due to more number of KA receptors. So durng lactation these part needs protection. Lactation stage protects these regions against adverse effect of KA administration. However pregnancy reduces the affinity of kainite receptors. The hormones of lactation down regulate kainite/

glutamate receptors and glial remodeling. Changes in the hippocampus of brain as a result of motherhood include dendroitic architecture, synaptic plasticity and decreased cell proliferation in the hippocampus during the lactation period. These changes maintain neuron expression of behavior and endocrine changes during lactation. Thus maternal brain goes through a series of adjustments that synchronize neuroendocrine, autonomic and behavioral responses which can be considered as a natural model for neuroplasticity.

Lactation represents a state in which internal signals trigger a system reorganization that is maintained by the afferent stimuli i.e. suckling and the adaptive efferent responses. Such reorganization might be demonstrable at the level of behavior, anatomy and physiology. Work on plasticity in the maternal brain has focused mainly on hypothalamic and limbic structures associated with the physiology of lactation, expression of maternal behavior and the stress response as depicted in figure.

Role of hormones in neuroprotection

High doses of progesterone reduce seizures and damage to the hippocampus. Progesterone and/or its metabolites might play an important role in the neuroprotective effects of lactation since this hormone is elevated for a significant period of time during pregnancy. Physiological or supraphysiological levels of estrogen reduce neuronal cell death from seizures. Estradiol and progesterone can reduce the neurotoxic effects of glutamate on the hippocampal region of the brain. Several studies have shown downregulation of caspase-3 expression and upregulate expression of antiapoptotic proteins of Bcl-2 family by 17-β estradiol. Oxytocin triggers uterine contraction and milk ejection in dairy animals. Oxytocin improve memory and learning process by developing long-lasting connection in neuron of hippocampus. It reduces stress-induced c-fos expression in dorsal hippocampus.While prolactin stimulates milk secretion in the mammary gland, prolactin is released in the CNS in response to suckling or milking stimulus. Prolactin hormone promotes maternal behavior, grooming, anxiolytic and neuroprotective actions.

❑❑❑

Chapter-20

Milking Behaviour

Temperament of the cows or buffaloes has been investigated in relation to milking behavior and milk yield. Temperamental cows and buffaloes have more milking time, less milk flow rate and less milk yield in comparision to docile animals. The primiparous cows are more temperamental at milking than the mulptiparous cows. The temperament of Sahiwal, Murrah buffaloes and crossbred cows at milking gradually declines and becomes normal in milking parlors within 15-20 days postpartum. More temperamental or wilder cattle have greater stress hormones level, decreased growth rates and average daily gain. These animals have poor immune response to pathogens. For example, the stress response is produced to help an animal to evade a predator as it activates the fight-or-flight response. This action increase the chances of survival of the animal. In contrast, the stress response to handling during management procedures may be harmful, as it may cause the animal to injure itself or a worker. The elevated stress hormones may inhibit normal physiological functions in reproduction and immunity. A rough handling during milking operations may be more stressful to the temperamental animal than docile and calmer. However, repeated handling may reduce the reaction responses.

It has been established that both hypothalamic-pituitary-adrenal axis and the sympathetic nervous system play important role in the body's response to stressors. Stress is currently defined as "a state in which homeostasis is actually threatened. In response to stressful stimuli, higher brain centers stimulate neurons in the paraventricular nucleus (PVN) of the hypothalamus, resulting in the synthesis and secretion of corticotrophin-releasing hormone (CRH) and vasopressin, VP (figure). Increased concentration of CRH and/or VP in the hypothalamic-hypophyseal portal blood induces release of anterior pituitary gland's corticotrophins which activate the adrenal axis. ACTH stimulates the production of glucocorticoids i.e. cortisol. In rodents the primary glucocorticoid is corticosterone. Glucocorticoids are released and distributed via circulatory system and act systemically to produce a variety of effects depending on (1) the amount of hormone secreted, (2) the duration of secretion, (3) the peripheral blood concentration of cortisol binding globulin, (4) the relative abundance of glucocorticoids receptors in the target tissue, (5) the tissue in which they exert their effect, and (6) the extent of excretion of glucocorticoid metabolites. Glucocorticoid is also responsible for negative feedback on both hypothalamus and pituitary by inhibiting synthesis and/or secretion of CRH, VP, and ACTH. Albumin is the major carrier protein for cortisol, but cortisol can also be transported by cortisol binding globulin (transcortin). Approximately 1-10% of cortisol circulates as a "free" steroid. Tissues also have the ability to increase or decrease available cortisol within cells through 11βhydroxysteroid dehydrogenase (HSD11β) enzymes, which convert cortisone to cortisol (type I) and vice versa.

The sympathetic nervous system is activated in response to many stressors often prior to stimulation of HPA axis. Upon stimulation, noradrenergic neurons in the brain and postganglionic sympathetic neurons innervating peripheral organs (e.g., heart, vasculature, kidneys, gut, and adipose) secrete norepinephrine into circulation, resulting in increased blood pressure, heart rate, and respiration rate. Additionally, nerve impulses in higher cortical centers within the brain relay messages through the limbic system resulting in the release of norepinephrine, serotonin, and acetylcholine which activate PVN. In conjunction with these actions, preganglionic sympathetic fibers innervating the adrenal medulla stimulate production and secretion of epinephrine and norepinephrine via acetylcholine.

An increase in epinephrine concentrations in the brain serves as an alarm system, resulting in a decrease in neurovegetative activities (eating and sleeping) and the activation of the stress response (HPA axis activation). The secretion of norepinephrine within the brain also activates the fear behaviors, enhances long-term memory and storage of adversely charged emotions in the hippocampus. The responses of HPA axis and the SMS to stress are highly coordinated. The activation of both the systems synergistically affect the response of each other. The release of norepinephrine, serotonin, and acetylcholine in the brain stimulate PVN resulting in the secretion of CRH. In this manner norepinephrine can modulate the release of ACTH and subsequently glucocorticoids.

High HPA activation in mice leads to increased size of adrenal, corticosterone and less immune response. High temperamental cattle have more cortisol and less live weight gain due to decreased feeding time and feed intake. Such animals have lower milk yield, protein, fat, conception rate, poor meat quality, high pH of carcass, reduced carcass weight and poor immune response.

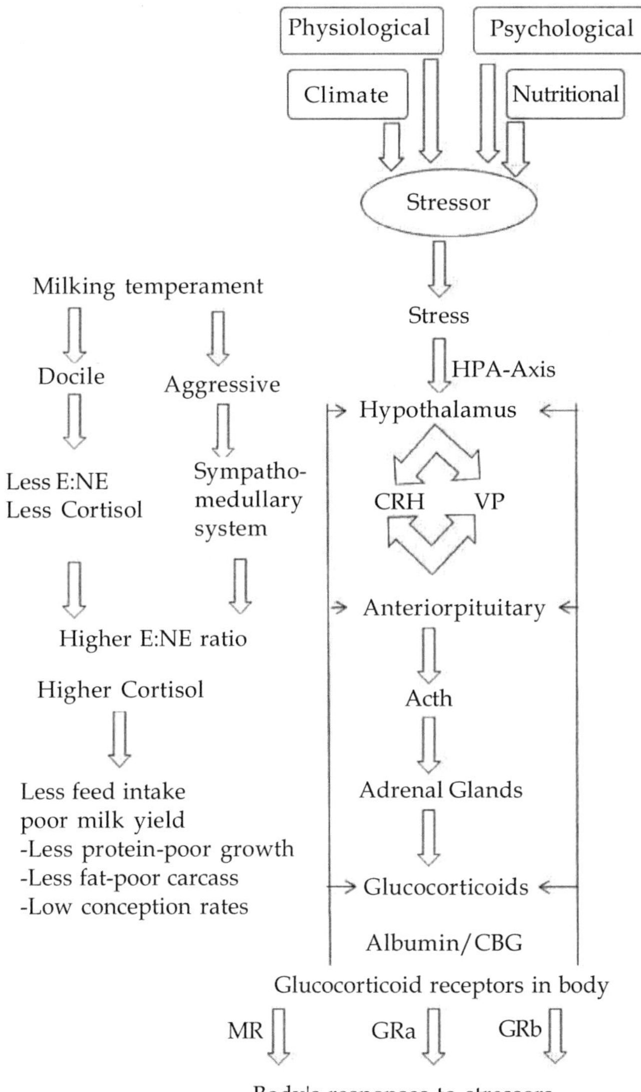

Figure. Milking temperament and stress induced hormone changes in dairy animals.

Chapter-21

Mitigation Strategies for Climatic Stress

Stress is a common term that is often associated with negative situations and settings. Climate change poses formidable challenge to the milk production potential of elite cows and buffaloes in India. The rise in ambient temperature together with increased precipitation and humidity aggravate the heat stress and adversely affect milk production and reproductive performance of dairy animals. The effect of extreme hot dry or hot humid weather is quite large and devastating for the low-income rural farmers due to substantial loss of milk production. Besides this, climate also has a negative impact on feed and fodder quantity and quality in summer season. India has become the largest milk producers in the word but livestock sector requires intensive and innovative tools to ameliorate climate stress in order to boost the milk production of lactating animals by 10-20 %.

Thermoneutral zone: The range of environmental temperatures over which the heat produced by a 'warm-blooded' animal remains fairly constant. Hence, it is the temperature range in which the animal is 'comfortable' and neither generate extra heat to keep body warm or spend metabolic energy on cooling mechanisms, such as panting. Animals adapted to cold environments tend to have broader thermoneutral zones than that of those living in hot environments.

Temperature humidity index

Temperature–humidity index (THI) is used to evaluate the combined effect of temperature and humidity. It is considered that at THI higher than 72, the animals would begin to suffer stress. To determine the heat stress, it is also important to determine the hours of stress during the number of days. As environmental temperature and the relative humidity increase, the loss of heat from the skin of cow diminishes and its corporal temperature increases (temperature of >25°C and humidity >70%). The animals move towards the wind, for a fresh or humid place or artificial shades to improve the comfort level. These mechanisms are necessary to maintain the normal body functions and reactions. The most productive, mature and heaviest animals are more susceptible to heat stress.

The upper critical temperature range for high producing exotic dairy cows and calves has been reported between 25 and 26°C. When animal can no longer dissipate enough metabolic heat to maintain homeothermy, vasodilation, sweating and panting mechanisms are invoked to dissipate the body heat. At this time, feed intake is also voluntarily reduced resulting in less heat generated by digestion and absorption of nutrients but energy requirementof maintenance increases with the temperature rising above (and below)18 to 20°C in exotic breeds. However, indigenous breeds of cows and buffaloes thrive well at 35°C due to adaptation and moderate milk production. Strategic planning of shelter management and feeding practices can mitigate heat stress to a great extent.

Effect on milk production and composition

Hot weather reduces milk production in cows having high genetic merit for milk production. With the extensive cross breeding, the average milk production per cow has doubled. Due to this reason, metabolic heat output per animal has increased substantially rendering animals more susceptible to heat stress. Numerous studies have examined the physiology, production, genetics,and management tools of heat stress, under both climatic laboratory and on-farm conditions. Lactating cows suffering from heat stress seek and remain in shade, reduce feed intake, drink more water, and show an immediate drop in daily milk yield.

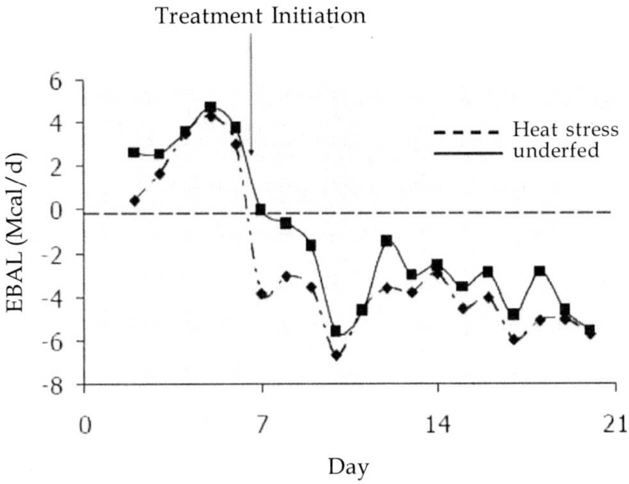

Figure. Effects of heat stress on calculated net energy balance in lactating Holstein cows. (Adapted from Wheelock *et al.*, 2006).

Table. Effect of seson on efficiency of milk production in cows

Attributes	Seasons	
	Summer	Winter
Body weight before experiment (kg)	408.3±20.5	409.0±12.7
Body weight after experiment (kg)	397.3±22.3	411.8±13.6
Body weight change (kg)	-11.0	±2.8
TDN consumed (kg)	6.63±0.17	9.42±0.37
D.E. of the feed (Mcal)	29.15±0.76	41.45±1.64
Energy for maintenance (Mcal)	12.55	12.55
Energy secreted in milk (Mcal)	6.45	9.44
Gross efficiency of milk production	22.13	22.77
Net efficiency of milk production (Without correcting for weight change)	41.35	33.84
Net efficiency of milk production (Corrected for weight change)	33.59	34.99

The milk production of the crossbred cows declines faster than the indigenous Sahiwal and Tharparkar cows. During hot dry season the drop in milk yield can be checked effectively, if crossbred cows are offered *ad lib* green fodder and water. Elite cows and buffaloes cannot withstand rigors of high ambient temperature and humidity leading to a significant reduction in milk yield (20-30 %) due to decline in the metabolic hormones, feed intake and increased respiration, pulse rate and body temperature. Somatic cell counts and incidence of mastitis rise due to unhygienic conditions during hot humid climate. However, it is unknown that how much milk yield is reduced due to hot conditions and how much improvement in management, nutrition and health could overcome the reduced production.

Methods to mitigate heat stress

1. Shelter management

Shelter is a prerequisite for the expression of full genetic potential of animal's production. Shelter management under normal condition has no meaning for the small and landless farmers as latter have no priority of animal shelter due to the lack of resources. One of the best ways of mitigating the heat stress is to keep the animals under trees or in mud houses, which is a very old and traditional practice in rural areas. But this practice is feasible only to a limited number of cows and buffaloes producing medium and low milk yield. The provision of tress in a loose housing system provides effective cooling against heat stress by lowering the ambient temperature (Up to 4 °C).

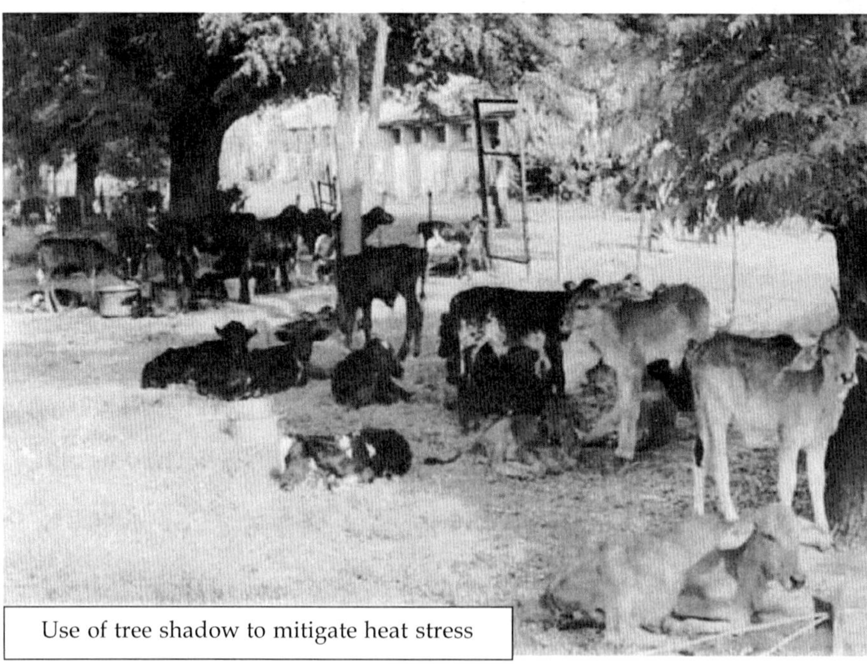

Use of tree shadow to mitigate heat stress

Many types of shelters made of bamboos with paddy straws/ thatch roof are being used by farmers. Such houses are quite economical and comfortable during hot dry and hot humid seasons. The use of paddy straw bedding (6 inches) over the asbestos roof of the animal shed during summer season reduces the heat stress and improves the milk yield of cows. Use of sand bedding and fan in hot dry and hot humid climate is also effective and economic way of minimizing the heat stress.

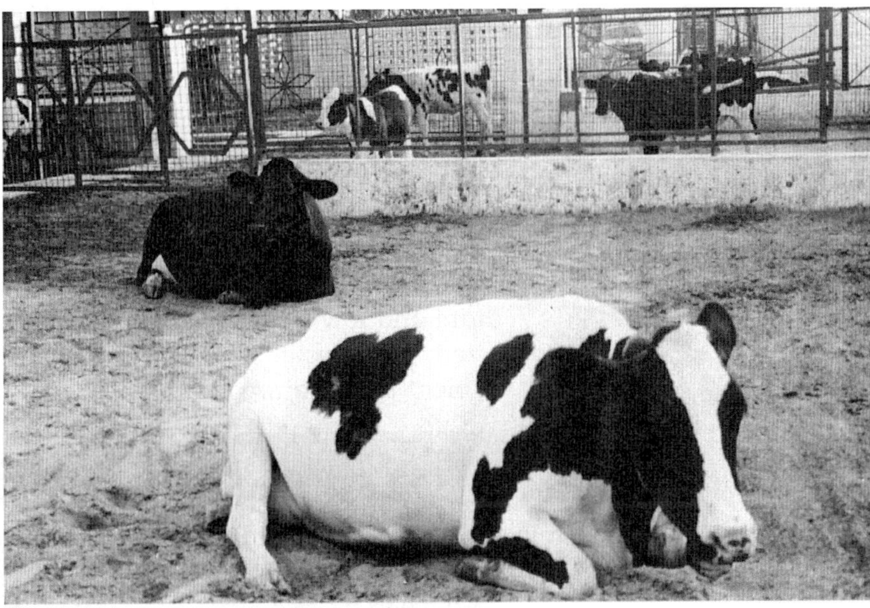

Photo: Use of sand bedding to alleviate stress of summer

2. Mist and water showers

Successful cooling strategies for lactating dairy animals are based on maximizing available routes of heat exchange by convection, conduction, radiation and evaporation. Provision of fans, wetting the animal's body surface, high pressure mist to cool the air in the animal shed and the facilities designed to minimize the transfer of solar radiation (i.e. use of sprinklers and thatch material over the roof of the shed) are used for heat abatement. Due to more awareness and ever increasing population density in urban areas, the progressive farmers now keep elite cows in the group of 50 or more. In such farms, summer induced dramatic decline in milk yield could be checked effectively by using mist or shower system.

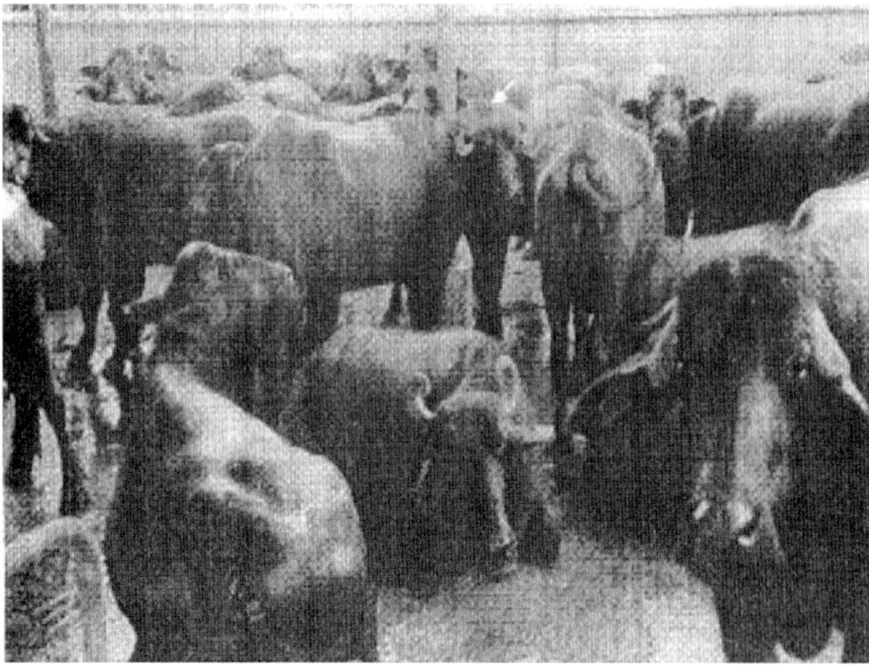

Water shower treatment durng summer

The efficacy of the mist system may be improved further by the use of fans. These systems have been shown to decrease the losses in milk yield and mortality in post-parturient cows. It also improves the reproductive performance (services/conception, conception rate, reduce days open) and DMI. Cooling pre-parturient dairy cows with shades, fans, and sprinklers when compared with sprinklers alone improved the total milk production of 60 days by 84.3 kg/cow and increased the profitability per cow. Excessive moisture in the ground or bedding of dairy cattle affects the behavior and physiology in many ways. Rainy or wet conditions drastically reduce the time of lying down in dairy cattle. They spend more energy while walking in the muddy and wet conditions with a reduction in feed intake. The wallowing of buffaloes is more effective than the water shower cooling during summer season. The lack of cleanliness associated with wet environments affects health conditions in dairy cattle including an increase in uterine and intra-mammary environmental pathogens that predispose dairy cattle to endometritis. Lameness is one of the most costly diseases on dairy farms and wet conditions contribute to softer hooves and an increase in lameness. Though cost of mist system installation is met within 3 months time period and farmers get a reasonable profit through its use. Another important constraint in the rural and peri-urban area is the availability of water. However, some measures are to be taken to recycle the used water in the mist cooling system. The dampness of floor renders the micro-environment favorable for the growth of the bacteria causing mastitis and thus hygiene needs to be maintained for better udder health. Short term experiments in crossbred cows have indicated no adverse effect of using the mist and fan system on udder health but long term effects on health and production needs to be investigated. The progressive farmers are using fan and mist system nowadays to mitigate heat stress. Mist cooling in hot humid season decrease milk temperature, udder skin temperature and skin temperature of the body effectively (figure). However, fan is effective only in the hot humid climate for better evaporative cooling in comparison to hot dry condition.

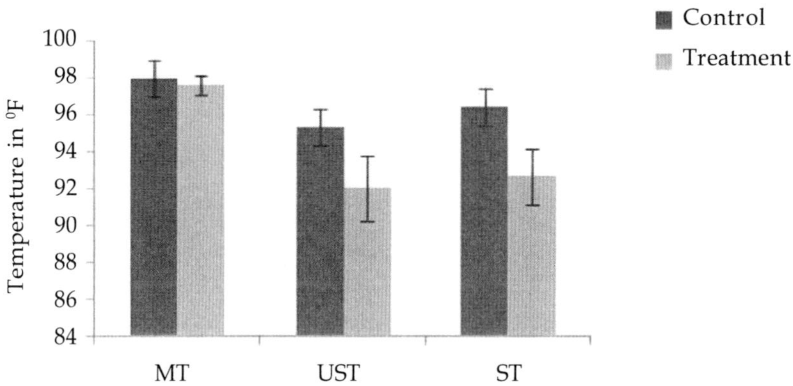

Figure. Dirunal variation in milk temperature, udder skin temperature and skin temperayure in lactating Murrah buffaloes during the hot humid season

Table. Mean ± S.E. of Thyroxine, triiodothyronine, insulin and cortisol levels in shower and wallow buffaloes during hot-dry and hot-humid season.

Parameter	Hot-dry		Hot-humid	
	Water shower	Wallowing	Water shower	Wallowing
Thyroxine (ng/ml)	50.65±0.50	52.57±0.67	48.25±0.54	50.57±0.61
Triiodothyronine (ng/ml)	1.97±0.03	1.88±0.03	1.83±0.04	1.99±0.03
Insulin (μU/ml)	8.30±0.26	10.86±0.27	7.86±0.33	9.62±0.30
Cortisol (ng/ml)	4.80±0.14	2.60±0.08	4.33±0.16	2.64±0.32
Milk yield (kg)	7.6±0.1	8.6±0.1	6.9±0.2	7.8±0.2
Feed intake (kg)	39.3±0.5	43.9±0.8	40.8±0.8	45.0±0.5

3. Feeding management

Energy is one of the most important requirements for milk synthesis and secretion. Heat stress reduces both feed intake and milk yield. The decline in nutrient intake has been identified as a major cause of reduced milk synthesis however, the exact contribution of declining feed intake to the overall reduced milk yield remains unknown. Feed intake and rate of passage of ingesta decreases at high ambient temperature and animal's water intake increases. The heat stress also alters the animal behavior and cows prefer to have their feed during nights when temperature decline. Night feeding during cool hours increases feed intake of cows. Heat-stressed cows had an immediate reduction (5 kg/d) in dry matter intake (DMI) with the decrease reaching nadir at day 4. Reduction in DMI can only account for 40-50 % of the decrease in milk production when cows are heat-stressed and about 50-60 % can be explained by other heat-stress induced changes.

During summer, feeding of total mixed ration or TMR (concentrate mixture+ straw +water) improves DMI, milk yield and meets the water requirements of animals. High feed intake by elite cows results in higher metabolic heat increment which requires effective thermoregulatory mechanisms to maintain body temperature in a thermoneutral zone and in physiological homeostasis. Cows can succumb to hyperthermia, if they fail to maintain thermoneutrality. Accurate measurement of time when cows enter heat stress is complicated because the responses to heat stress affect not only the energy balance but also water, sodium, potassium and chlorine metabolism. Water, sodium, potassium and chloride are important constituents of sweat and sweating is a major thermoregulatory mechanism used to dissipate excess body heat. Due to high metabolic heat increment especially during warm months, high-producing dairy cows may enter heat stress much earlier than their low-producing counterparts.

4. Hormone release

Climate has a major effect on endocrine profile due to alteration in metabolism. The release of hormones is controlled by the hypothalamus which is affected by high ambient temperature through input signals of cold and warm receptors. The basal metabolic rate, feed intake and the thyroxine release is increased at low tmeprature.

Cold stress stimulates thermo-sensitive cells in the anterior hypothalamus and affects secretion of glucocoroticoids. Growth hormone concentration increase in rats, but no seasonal variation occurs in GH level of cows. During short photoperiod, plasma prolactin levels decline and the water intake also decrease. It is considered that PRL is involved in water osmoregulation. Epinephrine and nor-epinephrine secretion increase due to change in deep body temperature that influences both neural and hormonal thermoregulatory mechanism (non-shivering thermogenesis). The mode of action is probably via the eyes signals to the pineal gland which in turn influence secretion of hormones. The secretion of prolactin is consistently elevated by long days during summer due to increased photoperiod which plays an important role in water and electrolyte metabolism. The increased water intake increases prolactin secretion. Growth hormone and insulin are unaffected by day length, whereas effects of day length on thyroxine and corticosteroids has not been clearly elucidated. Thyroid hormone, glucocorticoids, epinephrine and nor-epinephrine hormones decline at high ambient temperatures whereas aldosterone concentration increases to conserve sodium at the expense of potassium. The cortisol level increases initially in response to high ambient temperature but decline subsequently during long term exposure. Milk temperature and somatic cell count increase with increasing environmental temperatures in summer. Milk growth hormone concentration also increases with lactation level and declines significantly during summer heat stress. It has been elucidated that milk temperature and PRL level may serve as indicators of the impact of the climatic stress on lactating cattle.

5. Blood glucose

Mammary gland requires glucose to synthesize milk lactose, a primary osmoregulator of milk yield. However, at high ambient temperature, body (primarily skeletal muscle) utilizes glucose at an increased rate to generate less metabolic heat. As a consequence mammary gland may not receive adequate amounts of glucose; thus mammary lactose production and subsequent milk yield are reduced. This may be the primary reason for the additional reductions in milk yield that cannot be explained by decreased feed intake alone. Heat-stressed cows require special attention with regards to heat abatement and dietary considerations (concentrate: forage ratio and $HCO3^-$). Cows also have an extra requirement for dietary or rumen-derived glucose precursors. During heat stress, propionate is primarily converted into glucose by the liver. Highly fermentable starch diet, such as grain feeding increases rumen propionate production. Although propionate is the primary glucose precursor for lactose synthesis but feeding additional grains can be risky and may lead to rumen acidosis.

6. Nutritional amelioration

The average body weight of dairy cows has increased over the time as elite cows have been selected to produce more milk. Larger cows have larger gastrointestinal tract that allow them to consume and digest more feed. This in turn provides more nutrients for milk synthesis. The lactating cow uses ME for milk production at an average efficiency (q) of 65%. Heat increment (HI) during milk synthesis is also dependent upon the quality and quantity of feed that the animal consumes. On roughage diets, rumen fermentation yields a large molar excess of acetate compared with propionate and if the latter is insufficient to provide enough $NADPH_2$ then acetate may need to be converted, by some form of futile cycle to heat in order to prevent a metabolic excess. On a concentrate diet the molar proportion of propionate increases than that of acetate and so supply of $NADPH_2$ is not rate limiting. Thus increased milk production is related to elevate HI. Total milk production and HI has increased over time, although the rate of HI increase has been slower than of milk production.

The biological mechanism by which heat stress impact production and reproduction performance could be explained by the reduced feed intake, altered endocrine status, reduction in rumination and nutrient absorption and increased maintenance requirements resulting in a net decrease in energy availability for production. Reduction in energy intake during heat stress result into negative energy balance in lactating cows. Such cows largely depend on nonesterified fatty acids (NEFA) for energy. Despite having much greater energy content, oxidizing fatty acids generates more metabolic heat (about 2 kcal g or 13% on an energetic basis) as compared to glucose. Hence precursors for gluconeogenesis such as amino acids and propionate demand are greater.

Supplementation of excess protein aggravates the situation during periods of heat stress as protein itself is calorigenic and nitrogen excretion requires energy. Hence diet needs to be balanced for amino acids to prevent the feeding of excess crude protein. Recent advances in animal nutrition, including the feeding of ruminally-protected fats and protected proteins are among other endeavours to reduce metabolic heat production and supply the correct profile of nutrients to high producing cows in early lactation. Supplemental fat as rumen-inert fat, is used as an effective source of energy with low heat increment on straw-based diets in tropical environment. The feeding of prill fat or any other form of bypass fat enahnces postpartum milk production peroformance by improving the DMI, body weight, GH levels and decrease of NEFA, BHBA. Improvement in early onset of cyclicity and conception rate with less number of service per conception has also been found. An adequate supply of nutrients must also include well-balanced mixture of dietary minerals, especially of Na, K, Cl. These play a pivotal role in the thermal physiology of the cow and are influenced by the heat stress.

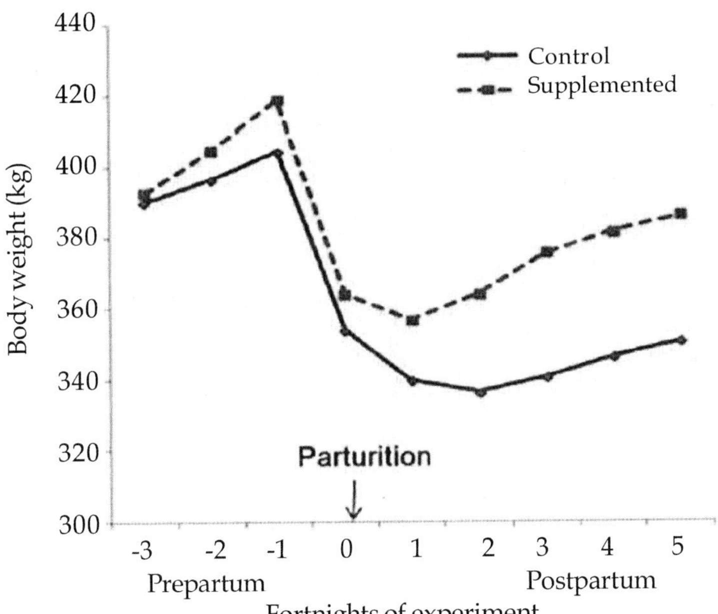

Figure. Body weight changes in control and prill fat supplemented cows

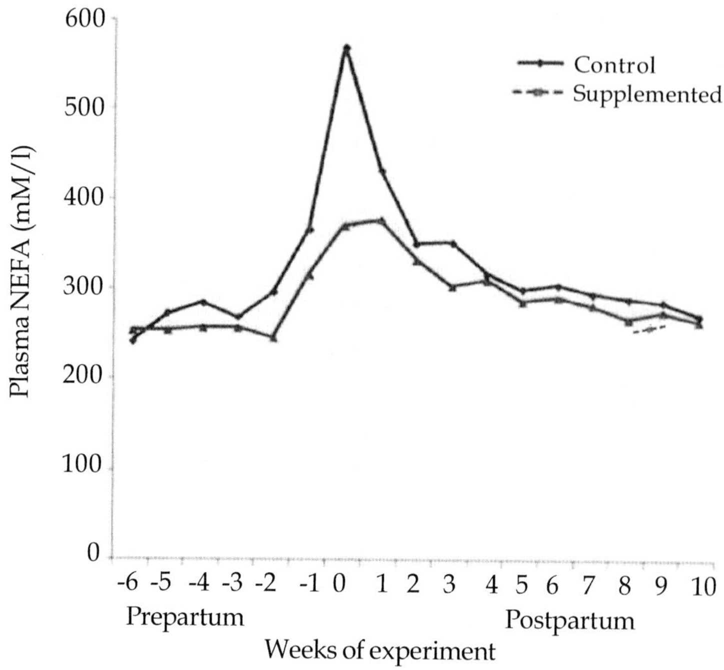

Figure. Plasma NEFA levels (μM/L) in control and prill fat supplemented cows

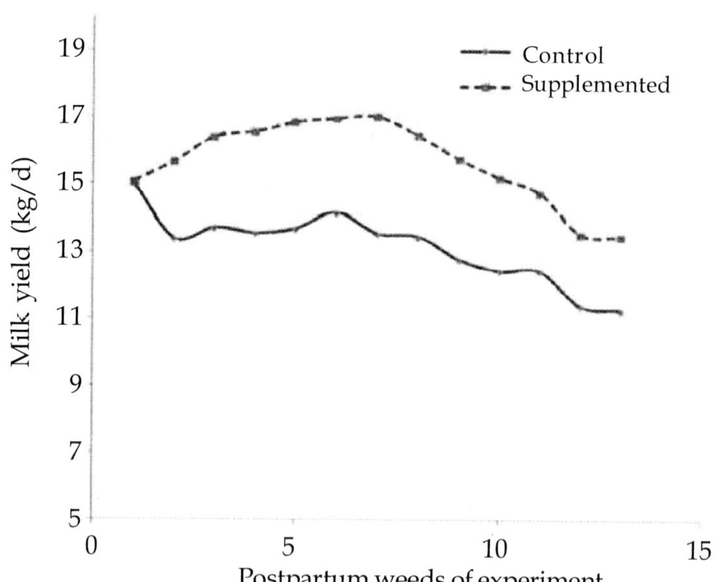

Figure. Milk yield changes in control and prill fat supplemented cows

Rumen protected protein and prill fat produced from oilseeds/ palm oil provide a practical feeding strategy to regulate nutrient partitioning. Feeding of prilled fat augment overall productivity of cows and buffaloes with increased milk yield (15-20%), however fat content vary. The postulated mechanism has been presented in figure. Feeding of 1 kg formaldehyde-treated oilseed protein meal supplement increased milk yield by 10% as compared with untreated protein meal supplements group in Indian cows and buffaloes fed on straw based diets. Improving productivity in dairy animals exposed to adverse environmental conditions may be achieved by improving the micro-environment around the animals and improving their nutritional management. Feeding of non-hormonal substances like choline chloride and milkofeed could be used to prevent decline in milk yield in summer season.

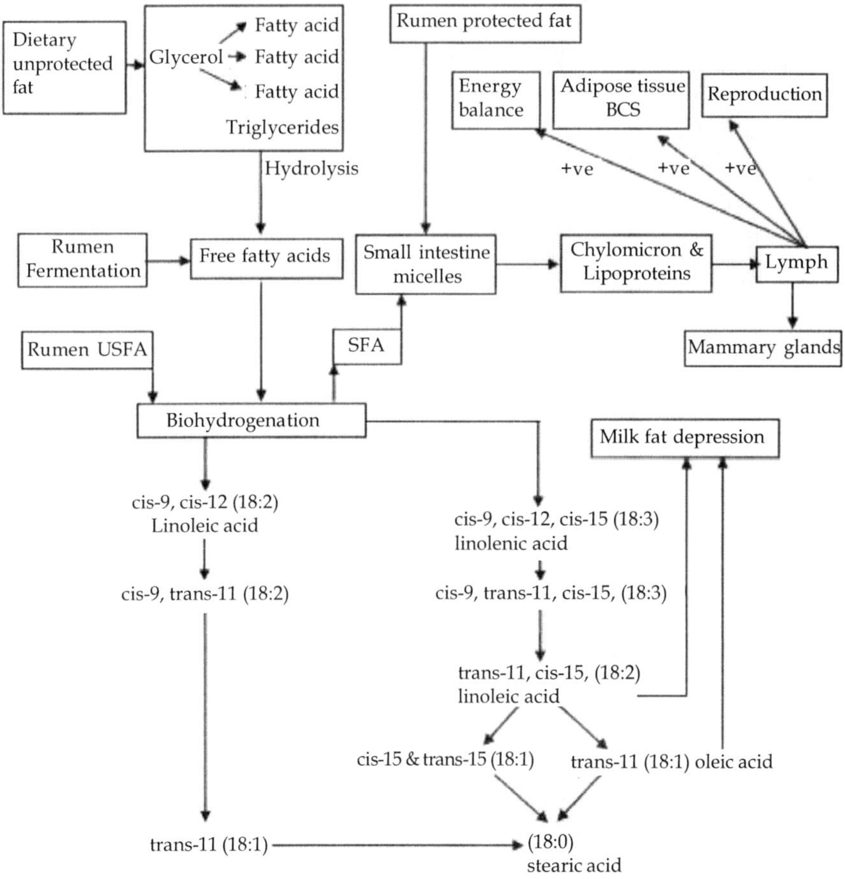

Figure. Metabolism of protected and unprotected fat in ruminants

7. Stress response pathways

Stress on animal and human beings occur in response to a stressor in different ways. Any stressor results in the release of nor-epinephrine hormone in the body to counter the challenge and therefore the "fight" hormone predominantly released are nor-epinephrine. If the intensity of stress arousal increases and a possible loss of control are felt by the individual, then epinephrine which is another "flight or anxiety" hormone is released. When stress is prolonged and seen as hopeless, the individual becomes more distressed and defeated. This activates the hypothalamus in the brain resulting in the final release of cortisol, a steroid hormone that is produced from the cortex of the adrenal glands. Fasting, food intake, exercising, awakening, psychosocial and climatic stressors causes the body to release cortisol. Animal and human studies have demonstrated that cortisol injections are associated with increased appetite, cravings for sugar, and weight gain. Cortisol indirectly influences appetite by regulating CRH (corticotrophin releasing hormone), leptin, and neuropeptide Y (NPY) released during stress. Fight or "flight" stress responses cause the heart to beat faster and harder as well as release more free fatty acids into the blood and suppress the immune system.

8. Cold stress

Lactating animals are more vunerable to heat stress than the cold stress. The following factors affect an animal's ability to withstand the cold climatic conditions.

- **Acclimation:** Cattle do adjust or acclimate to colder weather by growing a longer and thicker coat. This provides additional insulation against cold weather. The coat must be clean and dry to provide maximum protection to the cow. Dirt or moisture on the coat reduces its insulation value dramatically.
- **Fat layer:** Cattle in good condition with a thick fat layer is able to withstand the cold better than the thin cattle. The fat layer acts as another insulating layer between the animal's core and the environment.
- **Metabolic rate:** Cows increase their metabolic rate to enhance heat production to maintain body temperature. This increases the need for dietary energy so appetite is usually increased and cows eat more.

Hypothermia occurs when the body temperature drops well below normal. Mild hypothermia occurs with a body temperature of 30°C–32°C, moderate hypothermia range at 22°C–29°C and severe hypothermia incidence occurs below 20°C. As rectal temperature drops below 28°C, cows are not able to return to normal temperature without assistance through warming and the administration of warm fluids. As hypothermia progresses, metabolic and physiological processes slow down and blood is diverted from the extremities to protect the vital organs. Teats, ears and testes are prone to frostbite. The Cows are subjected to an environmental temperature below their lower critical temperature, without obvious signs of hypothermia. This increases the maintenance energy requirement of these animals as they adjust to these conditions and divert more energy to maintain body temperature.

Management factors to limit the effects of cold stress

- Monitor the weather conditions, minimum and maximum ambient temperature, increase the feeding quantity and frequency in response to cold weather. Late pregnant cows require additional grain feeding when the effective temperature falls below the lower critical level.
- Protect animals from cold wind as latter markedly reduces the effective temperature and increase cold stress on animals.
- Lactating animals may be provided with the paddy straw dry bedding (of 6 inches) which keeps warmness against the ground floor and increase the ability of cattle to withstand cold stress.
- Keep cows clean and dry so that the effect of cold weather is reduced. Wet coats greatly reduce insulating properties and make cows more susceptible to cold stress. Mud-caked coats also reduce the insulating properties of the hair.
- Provide additional feed like hay (wheat/paddy straw) and grain which help in the heat production and sufficient energy to animals to withstand the cold stress.
- Provide ample water available at all times. Limiting water will restrict the feed intake and make it more difficult for cows to meet their energy requirements. Excessively cold water may seriously limit the water intake.
- All efforts should be made to reduce the effects of cold stress on cows. This will help to reduce costs and improve production efficiency.

❏❏❏

Chapter-22

Partitioning of Nutrients in Lactating Animals

Mammary gland is one of the most highly differentiated and metabolically active tissues in the body and lactation is much more energy expensive than the pregnancy. Remarkable changes in partitioning of nutrients and metabolism takes place with the initaiton of lactation to meet out the increased demands of nutrients in mammary gland. The capacity of the cow to produce milk is determined by i) growth and development of mammary gland before and during pregnancy, and ii) animal's ability to supply the precursors for milk synthesis. It is still not clear which of these factors is more important for maximum milk production. The improved milk yield in early and mid lactation is associated with a proportionately greater partitioning of nutrients towards mammary gland at the expense of body reserves. Around parturition fetal calf requires only 1 % of the dam's energy intake while milk synthesis requirement may exceed upto 80 % of the net energy intake during early lactation. Cows producing very high peak milk yield (40 kg/d) exhibit mean decit of about 10 MCal NE/d during 2nd wk of lactation and 425 Mcal NE/d during the first 10 wks of lactation. This requirement is much more and exceeds than the maintenance requirement of the animals. Thus there is a shift in the partitioning of nutrient for a particular physiological stage and mammary gland gets priority for the purpose of milk synthesis. This mechanism of shift in nutrients towards mammary gland is called *Homeorhesis* which is different form homeostasis, (maintenance of internal environment of body). Kennedy introduced the term homeorhesis in his review on the thermoregulation. Both homoeostasis and homeorhesis are required to maintain the physiological and metabolic equilibrium.

Homeostasis - Maintenance of physiological equilibrium, i.e. constant conditions in the internal environment of body.

Homeorhesis- Orchestrated changes for the priorities of a physiological state, i.e. coordination of metabolism in various tissues to support a physiological state that could be growth, pregnancy or lactation. The Greek derivation of homeorhesis means "uniform-flow".

Change in nutritional environment	Genotype
	Genetic drives
Homeostatic partitioning	Telophoreltic/homeorhesis partitioning
Maintenance of physiological balance	Channel resources to different life functions
Alter partition of output to accommodate	Partition as per genetic drives

Figure. Homeostatic and teleophoretic nutrient partitioning (Friggens and Newbold, 2007)

Lactogenesis signals the shift from 'uterine nutrient transfer to foetus' to 'neonatal nourishment' at the mammary gland. Thus at partitioning, the mammary gland achieves metabolic priority over other tissues to perform the synthesis and secretion of milk. The nutrients deficient in feed are met by partitioning the nutrients from body reserves towards mammary gland. The increased energy demand of milk synthesis is regulated by modification in metabolism, endocrine and nervous system. Metabolic changes channelize more nutrients towards mammary gland. In early lactation the peak milk yield preceded by maximum dietary intake by several weeks leading to a state of energy deficit. The increased feed consumption contributes to nutrient pool in which plasma volume increase and total pool of nutrients also increase. However, energy losses occur through urine, feces, gases and heat production. The excess nutrients of metabolizable pool are deposited in adipose tissue, bone and muscle. There is a mobilization of nutrients from the body reserves due to negative energy balance when nutrient requirement is more and supply is limited.

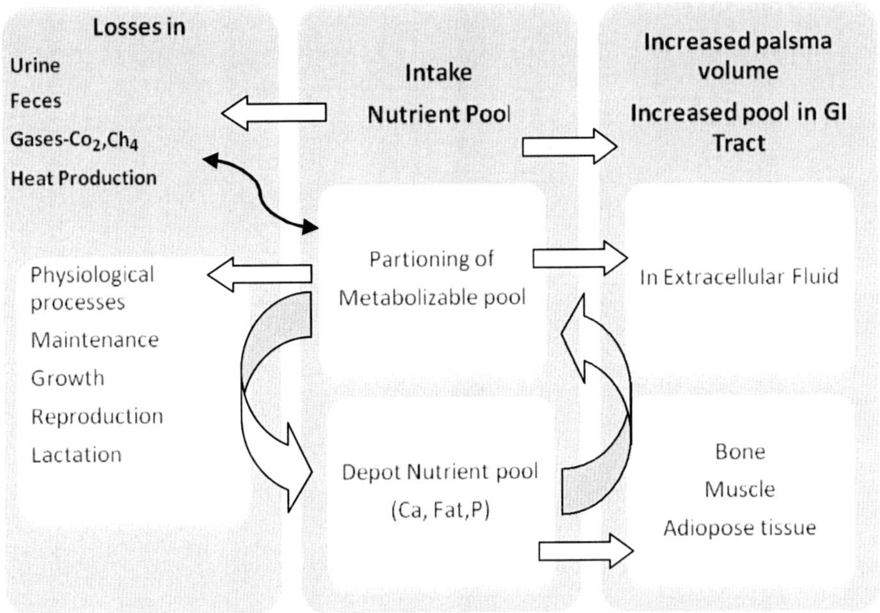

Fig. Mechanism of partitioning of nutrients

Metabolic adaptation during lactation

Feed and water intakes: Lactogenesis signals drain of massive nutrient from dam to support the growth of calf. Hypothalamic feed and water intake centers are stimulated by suckling or milking stimuli resulting in more feed and water intake. In addition digestive adaptation like hypertrophy of GI tract, increased rate of passage of ingesta, increased blood flow and nutrient flow across GI tract take place. Thus lactating animal consumes more feed and water to meet the energy requirement of milk synthesis. Partitioning of nutrients is further attenuated by increase in cardiac output, higher metabolic activity of epithelial cell, more transport of nutrients from blood to mammary gland and change in endocrine profile. The increased requirement of electrolyte (NaCl) develops cravings for "*salt drive*".

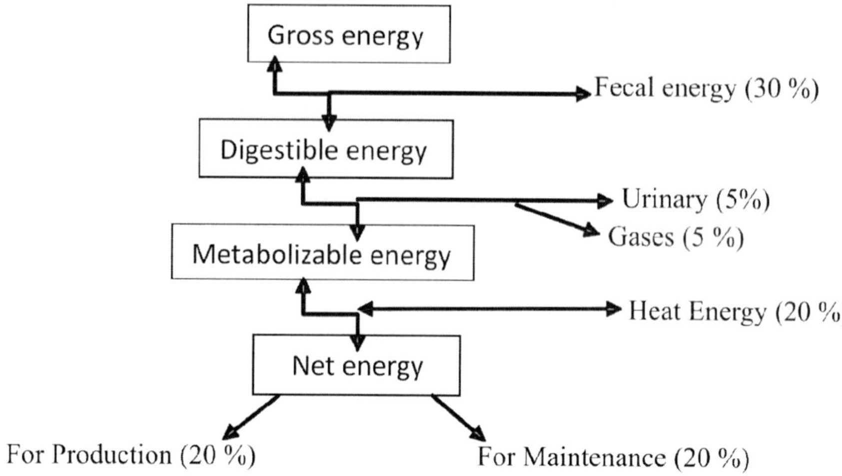

Partitioning of energy for production and maintenance in animals

All these changes accommodate the increased demand of the nutrients for milk synthesis.

Resting energy expenditures of young adults can be estimated by following formula.

Heat production = 70 kcal/day x $W^{*0.75\ kg}$

Since Net energy, (NE) is Maintenance energy (ME) minus heat energy, the efficiency of ME utilization will influence availability of NE. During peak lactation, and for several weeks after peak lactation, the metabolism of the high-yielding dairy cow is orientated to meet the demands of udder. Fat is utilized with greater efficiency than protein due to energy cost of urea production. In mature adult animals energy is stored as fat. Mobilization of fat reserves during period of peak lactation result in negative energy balance (NEBAL) because of low energy content of feed. When body reserves are exhausted the milk production declines. Maintenance and pregnancy requirement are met at the expense of lactation and growth. During this period changes occur in most areas of intermediary metabolism and all of these changes are to a greater or lesser extent, coordinated and integrated by the cow's endocrine system.

Water intake

Water is the main component of milk and contribute to 34 -89 % of total volume of milk in different species. Lactating animals consume more water as it is important for milk secretion. Increased water intake by the mammary gland triggers thirst drive in animals. To compensate this drive, water intake of animal and its flow and absorption in GI tract increases. ADH is released due to suckling or milking stimulus in lactating animals. Deficiency of water stimulates ADH secretion which enhances water reabsorption from kidney tubule.

Lipid metabolism

Fat is the major component as it supplies more percentage of calories in milk. The source of milk fat could be from de-novo synthesis from acetate or uptake of fatty acid precursors from blood. Metabolic adaptations lead to increase in lipolysis and decreased lipogeneis in liver. To meet the increased energy requirement, mobilization from fat depot, bone muscle takes place during early and peak lactation. Mammary gland utilizes free fatty acids for the energy and fat synthesis.

List of the metabolic changes associated with lactogenesis in ruminants

Physiological function	Metabolic changes
Milk synthesis	Increased use of nutrients by Mammary gland
Feed intake	Increased feed and water intake by stimulation of feed and water intake centers
Digestion	Increase in small and large intestine volume
	Increase in rate of passage of digesta
	Increase blood flow to GI tract
Lipid metabolism	Increased lipolysls
	Decreased lipogenesis in Adipose tissue
Glucose metabolism	Increased gluconeogenesis and
	Increased glycogenolysis in Liver
	Decreased use of glucose in body tissue and
	Increased use of lipid as energy source
Protein metabolism	Mobilization of protein reserves from Muscle and body tissue
	Increased uptake from GI tract
Mineral metabolism	Increased absorption and mobilization of calcium in kidney, liver, gut and bone

Glucose metabolism

Increased glucose requirements of gravid uterus during late pregnancy and of lactating mammary glands necessitate major adjustments in glucose production and utilization in maternal liver, adipose tissue, skeletal muscle and other tissues. As a result of this more nutrients are partitioned towards mammary gland. Ruminants rely principally on hepatic gluconeogenesis for their glucose supply. Hepatic glucose synthesis increases during late pregnancy and early lactation to accommodate uterine or mammary demands. These responses are mediated by reduced tissue sensitivity and responsiveness to insulin, decreased tissue expression of insulin-responsive glucose transporter (GLUT4). Peripheral tissue responses to insulin remain severely attenuated during early lactation but recover as the animal progresses through mid- lactation. Somatotropin has a predominant homeorhetic influence during lactation because exogenous administration of GH causes specific changes in glucose metabolism of various non-mammary tissues which mimic normal adaptations to early lactation. Ruminant has glucose sparing mechanism by decreasing the utilization of glucose for lactose synthesis, while acetate is used for fat synthesis and energy purpose. Absence of citrate cleavage pathway in mammary gland of ruminant and adipose tissue prevent utilization of glucose in fat synthesis. Thus acetate is being used as a source of energy and for fat synthesis, while glucose is spared for lactose synthesis. *Due to this reason, glucose does not contribute carbon unit for fatty acid synthesis in ruminants.* Ruminants utilize all the above alterations in glucose metabolism during lactation. *In non-ruminants, acetate is* very less in blood and does not participate in energy production and fat synthesis. The increase in food intake increases blood glucose level and the lactose synthesis in non-ruminant.

The calf can utilize glucose from lactose as rumen fermentation is delayed for few weeks. Once rumen start functioning, lactose does not escape rumen degradation. Since glucose is utilized for lactose synthesis and energy purpose, gluconeogenesis and glycogenolysis increases in liver so that more glucose is available.

Minerals and electrolytes metabolism

Calcium, phosphorus and potassium are the major minerals in milk. Their requirement is met mainly from dietary source or through mobilization from bones, gut, kidney and liver. Sodium level is less in milk as lactose is the main determinant of milk osmotic pressure. However, lactating animals develop *salt drive* during lactation due to increased requirement of sodium for transport of various nutrients through various nutrient pools and across the wall of GI tract. When dietary source is poor in Ca, P, K and Na, the increased demand of these minerals is met by more absorption from GI tract and increased mobilization. Lactating animals receive enough potassium from roughage and concentrate mixture. However, high yielding cows consume more concentrate ration than the roughage; therefore potassium supplementation may be required in high yielding cows. During heat stress, lactating animals secrete more K in sweat and should be supplemented with potassium. The concentration of Ca is also important as deficiency of it (< 5 mg %) lead to milk fever after parturition.

Protein metabolism

Low dietary protein and inadequate amino acids availability in feeds lead to mobilization of protein from the muscles and other body tissues. The amino acid requirements increases due to protein synthesis in lactation. The flow of amino acid across digestive tract also increases. The requirement of lysine and methionine is high for milk synthesis in cattle and these amino acids are considered rate limiting for milk protein syntheisis. Some nonessential amino acids (proline, glutamate-glutamine) also may become limiting during lactation because of their unique contributions to milk protein synthesis. During different phase of lactation, an ideal diet may be prepared for freshly calved animals to meet out production and reproduction requirement. Some of the nutritional points are highlighted below for the formulation of diet:

- Use different roughage and concentrate rations to fulfill dry matter and nutrients requirement
- Nutrients dense feed may be fed during early lactation
- Different nutritional technologies like bypass fat, bypass protein, chelated minerals feeding may be used at the time of formulating the diet
- Secretion rates and the plasma concentration of insulin and growth hormone could be altered by altering the feeding patterns like dietary roughage: concentrate ratio, frequency of feeding, proportion of undegradable dietary protein and physical form of the diet.

Mammary blood flow

The synthesis of milk is a continual process and is correlated to milk secretion. Cow's udder has prominent artery and vein during lactation due to increased blood flow which partitions the nutrients more through vascular bed of mammary gland relative to other tissues. Mammary gland of lactating animals receives more blood supply than the dry animals. Thus increased blood flow rate results in increased supply of nutrients to the mammary gland, increased secretary activity of mammary gland and increase in extraction efficiency of epithelial cells. All these changes are necessary for more synthesis of milk by the mammary gland. The increased blood flow to mammary gland is important from three points of view i.e. percent of total cardiac output being received by the mammary gland, extraction efficiency of mammary tissue and the total mammary gland blood flow. Increase in blood flow to the mammary gland may not have any effect on diverting nutrients, if cardiac output also increase as it increases blood flow to the other body tissues also. Similarly if extraction efficiency of epithelial cells decreases with increasing blood flow rate, there is no net gain in substrate uptake by epithelial cells (extraction efficiency). Mammary uptake of milk precursor is directly related to the requirement of that nutrient for milk synthesis. Mammary blood flow can be measured by methods like antipyrine technique, Evan blue dye method, electromagnetic flow meter, thermal detection and radioactive microspheres method. Mammary uptake can be measured by arterial and venous difference of a substrate or hormone.

Arterial flow- venous flow of a precursor (AV difference) = Arterial concentration- Venous concentration.

Mammary uptake = AV difference x Blood flow

The uptake of milk precursor by mammary gland is limited by rate of blood flow than by changes in extraction. The studies in cows and goat indicate little change in arterial-venous difference with low or high blood flow rate and with low or high substrate concentration. Certain vasodilator substances like bradykinin, acetylcholine and histamine cause vasodilation of blood vessels but their role in control of mammary blood flow is not known. However, increase in blood glucose concentration lowers mammary blood flow. Mammary blood flow also increases with increase in amount of secretary tissue. Dry and old animals have more resting blood flow than the younger ones. Mammary blood flow rate is correlated to milk yield during different stages of lactation. In early lactation, the ratio of mammary blood flow to milk yield is 1000 ml: 1ml, which decline to 400ml: 1ml in late lactation. The average ratio of blood flow rate to milk yield is 500:1ml.

Hormonal regulation of nutrient supply

Hormonal regulation is a function of concentration of circulatory hormones in blood and the number and affinity of hormone receptors. Both of these processes may themselves be hormonally regulated. Certain hormones like growth hormone, glucocorticoids and thyroid hormones can play both catabolic and anabolic roles depending upon the metabolic status of the animal and the physiological process considered. Unlike the situation in non-ruminants, blood glucose is not a significant source of carbon for ruminant milk fat synthesis. The primary gluconeogenic precursors in ruminants are-propionate (intestinal absorption), amino acids (intestinal absorption, proteolysis), glycerol (lipolysis) and lactic acid (intestinal absorption, muscle metabolism). Propionate is quantitatively the most important precursor for glucose during lactation. Results from studies in ruminants and non-ruminants suggest that insulin, glucagon, catecholamines and glucocorticoids are primarily responsible for regulating both the supply of gluconeogenic substrates and modulating the gluconeogenic pathway in the liver. There are two ways in which gluconeogenesis is promoted by glucagon and the catecholamines: both directly stimulate the process in liver causing rapid inactivation of L-type pyruvate kinase. For glucagon, the effect is mediated by cAMP and cAMP-dependent protein kinase, whereas catecholamines are released from nerve endings within the liver and operate via α- and β-adrenergic receptors. In addition, both enhance the supply of gluconeogenic and milk-fat precursors by mobilizing free fatty acids and glycerol from adipose tissue. Catecholamines stimulate lactate production from muscle.

During early lactation the concentration of glucocorticoids rises and then falls during later stages when milk yield falls. They enhance the action of insulin on lipogenesis and antagonise the action of insulin on glucose utilisation. They also help in gluconeogenesis. The glucocorticoids exert a permissive influence on both the lipolytic action of the catecholamines and other hormones and on the gluconeogenic effect of catecholamines and of glucagon at the liver. In addition, cortisol stimulates mobilization of amino acids from muscle. Thyroid hormones, thyroid stimulating hormone (TSH), adrenocorticotrophic hormone (ACTH) and the prostaglandins (PGFs) stimulate tissue mobilization (lipolysis), however, relative importance of these hormones in supplying the gluconeogenic and milk-fat precursors has yet to be established. Thyroid hormones and cortisol modulate nutrient partitioning toward milk production and visceral protein synthesis.

Growth Hormone

The action of growth hormone with respect to protein metabolism is anabolic i.e. it preserve the protein reserves particularly during energy deficiency by inhibiting proteolysis and stimulate the incorporation of amino acids into the tissues. As far as lipid metabolism is concerned, growth hormone stimulates lipolysis, and inhibits lipogenesis in the adipose tissues and subsequently stimulates the nutrient mobilisation, by diverting glucose and fatty acids away from tissue deposition towards mammary gland, during lactation. It has been reported that changes in growth hormone levels in blood are positively correlated with changes in milk yield.

The somatotropic axis is decoupled during early lactation resulting in dramatic elevations of plasma growth hormone concentrations without the expected rise in insulin-like growth factor-1 (IGF-I) secretion. Likewise, insulin sensitivity declines substantially from late gestation to early lactation. These endocrine shifts are critical for promoting the mobilization of stored nutrients and sparing glucose for use by the mammary gland. This conservation of glucose is particularly important in ruminants. GHR 1A expression partially coordinates the high milk production phenotype that typifies dairy cattle. After calving there is a decrease in liver GHR 1A mRNA that leads to low postpartum liver GHR expression. The loss of liver GHR causes a GH refractory state in liver and liver does not produce IGF-I in response to GH. This refractory state represents an uncoupling of GH - IGF-I axis that is caused by the inactivation of the GHR. The subsequent decrease in blood IGF-I concentration leads to diminished negative feedback and pituitary production of GH increases. Thus elevated postpartum GH supports milk production. However low-producing dairy cattle may not uncouple their somatotropic axis after calving. Despite generous and ad. libitum postpartum feeding, the somatotropic axis remain uncoupled until the demand of the mammary gland for nutrients is reduced (involution of the gland) or the capacity of the cow to consume nutrients (feed intake) increases. Greater nutrient intake and improved energy balance in later lactation leads to elevated insulin and a direct effect on the GH axis via the effects of insulin on GHR expression.

The recoupling of the axis (establishment of liver GHR) causes an increase in IGF-I that acts negatively on GH secretion. The increase in insulin and IGF-I and the decrease in GH switches the postpartum dairy cow from a catabolic state (low insulin, low IGF-I, and elevated GH) to an anabolic state (high insulin, high IGF-I, and low GH). The lower insulin and IGF-I concentrations theoretically reduce ovarian responsiveness to gonadotropins because there is a synergistic relationship between the IGFs and insulin with gonadotropins for a variety of cellular functions including mitogenesis and steroidogenesis. The synergism is caused by the ability of IGFs and insulin to increase gonadotropin receptor numbers and increase the activity of gonadotropin receptor second messenger systems.

Prolactin

Lactation results in an increase in serum prolactin, the primary lactogenic hormone. Several investigators have proposed that prolactin coordinates lipid metabolism in adipose and liver tissue to partition nutrients to the mammary gland. Blocking the release of prolactin during lactogenesis or in early lactation produces not only the negative effects on mammary synthesis of milk but also results in an increase in adipose and liver pathways of lipid synthesis as well as reduction in the rates of lipid mobilisation from adipose tissues.

Insulin

During early lactation serum insulin concentration falls in cows, and later recovers as lactation progress and milk yield declines. Insulin is the major anabolic hormone for promoting lipid synthesis and inhibiting lipolysis in adipose tissues, promoting protein synthesis and inhibiting proteolysis in muscle, stimulating glucose uptake by muscles, inhibiting gluconeogenesis in liver. Mammary cells from cow possess insulin receptors but insulin does not have a direct effect on mammary cells during lactation in cows, hence a fall in serum insulin have no deleterious effects on the mammary gland itself. Insulin appears to be required for the induction of lactogenesis in mammary tissues in cows and buffaloes.

Glucagon

Glucagon antagonises some actions of insulin. The serum insulin: glucagon ratio is thought to be important in the control of liver metabolism. Glucagon stimulates gluconeogenesis and glycogenolysis whereas insulin inhibits.

Catecholamines

Stimulation of sympathetic nervous system leads to the release of noradrenaline in adipose tissues which increases lipolysis and inhibits lipogenesis. Noradrenaline interacts with beta-receptors of the adipocyte resulting in the activation of hormone-sensitive lipase enzyme and hence increased lipolysis.

Leptin

In ruminants, leptin a protein hormone is secreted almost exclusively by white adipose tissue (WAT). Leptin acts predominantly on isolated regions of the brain, where it serves as satiety signal, as shown by hyperphagia of leptin-deficient humans and mice, and by reduced feed intake in leptin-treated animals, including ruminants. Plasma leptin is increased by adiposity and is higher in females than in males. Plasma leptin concentration is reduced rapidly during periods of under nutrition and may regulate neuroendocrine mechanisms responsible for the partitioning of energy. Plasma leptin remain constant at 2.3ng/ml until 1yr of age. Leptin may modulate mammary parenchyma development as leptin is reduced abruptly around the time of parturition in lactating dairy cows. The periparturient reduction in plasma leptin precedes significant depletion of lipid reserves, but coincides with the onset of negative energy balance, decreased plasma insulin and increased plasma growth hormone levels (GH). Current evidence indicates leptin involvment in the regulation of energy homeostasis. Low concentration of plasma leptin during under nutrition induces increased appetite as well as neuroendocrine adaptations responsible for metabolic adaptations and energy conservation. Insulin is a positivere gulator of plasma leptin in lactating dairy cattle when in positive energy balance. However, role of insulin and GH in regulating plasma leptin is still inconclusive in dairy cattle.

Leptin interacts with six types of receptors (Ob-Ra–Ob-Rf, or LepRa-LepRf) which in turn are encoded by a single gene, LEPR. Ob-Rb is the only receptor isoform that can signal intracellularly via the Jak-Stat and MAPK signal transduction pathways, and is present in hypothalamic nuclei. It is unknown whether leptin can cross the blood-brain barrier to access receptor neurons, because the blood-brain barrier is somewhat absent in the area of the median eminence, close to where the NPY neurons of the arcuate nucleus are present. It is generally thought that leptin might enter the brain at the choroid plexus, where there is intense expression of a form of leptin receptor molecule that could act as a transport mechanism. Once leptin has bound to the Ob-Rb receptor, it activates the stat3, which is phosphorylated and travels to the nucleus to effect changes in gene expression. One of the main effects on gene expression is the down-regulation of the expression of endocannabinoids, responsible for increasing appetite. There are other intracellular pathways activated by leptin, but less is known about how they function in this system.

The biology of leptin has been studied most extensively in the central nervous system for the regulation of food intake and energy balance. In recent years, a number of publications have reported leptin to be a hormonal factor that informs several hormonal circuits and biological peripheral functions of the nutrition status of the organism. Evidences have reported the role of leptin to regulate mammogenesis during a virgin, pregnancy and involution. In mammary gland, leptin exert also an autocrine and/or paracrine activity which affects the development of duct, formation of alveolus, expression of milk protein gene and onset involution of mammary gland. Plasma leptin is positively regulated by fatness and to a lesser extent by the plane of nutrition in dairy cattle at all stages of the lactation cycle. Plasma concentration of leptin remains highest during pregnancy and is reduced by 25 to 50 percent in periparturient dairy cows due to reduced plasma insulin suggesting that leptin participates in the regulation of metabolism in the periparturient dairy cows. An alternative hypothesis is that reducing fat leads to a reduction in circulating adipokines, such as leptin, that play a role in stimulating the hyperphagia in early lactation.

Leptin synthesis has been found in the placenta of both human and livestock animals suggesting a role in controlling growth of the foetus and neonate. Colostrum and milk contain high amounts of leptin, in particular during the first few days of lactation that cause a correlation between milk leptin and plasma leptin, body weight and body mass index. Furthermore, other studies suggest that milk leptin may control appetite. The few published papers report that leptin may be produced by different cell types in the mammary tissue, and may act as a paracrine factor on mammary epithelial cell proliferation, differentiation and/or apoptosis via adipose-epithelial and/or myoepithelial-epithelial cellular interactions. In addition to leptin synthesis, epithelial cells may transfer leptin from the blood, and these two mechanisms may account for the presence of leptin in the milk, however the respective parts of these two processes remain to be determined. If leptin levels in milk (and specially colostrum) are found to be significant, this hormone could be involved in neonate physiology.

Metabolic adaptation in organs during milk secretion

Liver and kidney

Liver is the major site of glucose production in dairy animals. Meeting the increased demand for glucose to synthesize lactose in mammary gland requires a two- to three fold increase in hepatic glucose production. Liver contains some reserves of glucose as glycogen but these are trivial compared with the need for glucose, hence the requirement of glucose is met by increased gluconeogenesis. This is achieved through three mechanisms:

- An increase in liver size although this appears to lag behind the increase in milk yield
- An increase in activity/unit weight of tissues arising from increased activity of gluconeogenic enzymes i.e. Glucose-6-phosphatase, Fructose-1, 6 diphosphatase, PEP Carboxykinase and Pyruvate carboxylase
- The pyruvate carboxylase arises from an increase in blood flow through the liver

Besides, an increase in propionate and amino acid absorption from gut and increased release of lactate by muscle and adipose tissues, glycerol release from adipose tissues and amino acid release from muscle can also be used for glucose synthesis. Estimates indicate that propionate supplies 32 to 73 per cent of the total glucose demand during lactation. The kidneys also make minor contribution to glucose production through gluconeogenesis. However, neither the size of the organ nor the activities of its key gluconeogenic enzymes alter with lactation. The liver is also major site of lipid metabolism. During early lactation, supply of fatty acid to the liver is increased as a result of a rise in the unesterified fatty acid concentration in the blood (due to increased lipolysis) and the increase in blood flow to the liver.

Adipose tissue

The physiological changes in dairy animals before parturition prepare the adipose tissues for the massive release of fatty acids, and accordingly the mammary gland is prepared for receiving the increased supply of nutrients. At parturition there is massive mobilisation of fatty acids from adipose tissues and consequently a dramatic rise in plasma free fatty acids. Simultaneously, there is a considerable increase in the activity of the enzyme lipoprotein lipase in the mammary gland, as a preparatory step for the cleaving long chain fatty acids from the circulating triglycerides. During the early part of lactation, adipose tissue witness a high rate of lipolysis and a very low rate of lipogenesis and the dairy animal is in negative energy balance. A cow in early lactation can even lose 20 to 50 kg of fat in 6 weeks.

Optimal nutrition is important to exploit dairy animals genetically for production and reproduction. Losing more fat from body reserve indicates suboptimum nutrition and thus an animal may not be able to show its full potential for milk production. In this way, a dairy farmer faces hidden losses in milk production. Also a healthy body condition is required for proper functioning of reproductive organs.

Skeletal muscle

A loss of skeletal muscle protein during lactation has been reported by many researchers. The limited available data suggest that this is primarily due to an increase in protein degradation with little or no fall in protein synthesis. Amino acids released from muscle are probably used either for protein synthesis in the mammary gland or gluconeogenesis in the liver. There is no fall in protein synthesis in muscle during lactation.

❑❑❑

Chapter-23

Role of Hypothalamus and Pineal Gland in Lactation

Hypothalamic regulation of prolactin secretion in animals and human being is alomost similar and regulated by prolactin inhibiting factor (PIF) and dopamine. Hypothalamic neuro-transmitters and polypeptides either inhibit or stimulate prolactin release. Pituitary stalks section or lesions in basal tuberal region of the hypothalamus increase prolactin release and may initiate lactation. There is some evidence that dopamine may account for most, if not all, of the prolactin release inhibiting activity of the hypothalamus. Agents that increase dopamine activity like L-dopa and monoamine oxidase inhibitors depress prolactin release. Acetylcholine inhibits prolactin release via catecholamines release.

Hypothalamus factors that stimulate prolactin release are polypeptide prolactin releasing factor (PRF), thyrotropin releasing hormone (TRH) and serotonin. TRH is as effective in releasing prolactin as in releasing TSH, but under most physiological states, TSH and prolactin release do not occur together. Serotonin and its precursors, tryptophan and 5-hydroxytryptophan, are powerful releasors of prolactin and have been shown to be involved with prolactin release during suckling, stress etc. Other agents in the hypothalamus that can stimulate prolactin release include GABA and some prostaglandins, but these have not yet been shown to be involved in physiological control of prolactin secretion. Exteroceptive stimuli that alter prolactin release act through the CNS and hypothalamus.

Role of pineal gland in lactation

The significance of the pineal gland secretion on the mammalian reproductive system has been extensively studied. However, comparatively less work has been done on a possible impact of the pineal on lactation. Pineal gland secretes two important hormones-melatonin and serotonin. Administration of melatonin and serotonin lower peak milk yield curve in rabbits but have no inhibitory effect on lactation in rats. Supplemental lighting and bovine pineal extract can alter lactation in the mouse. Infusion of melatonin (20 μg/h, s. c.) daily into these goats either for 8 h (the long-day-type infusion) or for 16 h (the short-day-type infusion) to mimic the nocturnal profile of plasma melatonin under long days or short days, respectively. The long-day-type melatonin infusion for 9 days, in comparison with control saline infusion, accelerated prolactin secretion, inducing a nocturnal rise in plasma prolactin; which was comparable to that seen in the pineal intact goats under long photoperiods. On the other hand, the short-day-type melatonin infusion suppressed prolactin secretion throughout the day as the short-day treatment did in intact goats. The prevailing photoperiod appeared to have no distinct effect on these prolactin responses to exogenous melatonin. The results indicate that the information about external light-dark cycles is converted by the pineal gland into the endocrine signal as a daily pattern of melatonin secretion, which eventually regulates prolactin secretion from the pituitary gland of the goat.

Seasonal rhythm of prolactin secretion is under pineal control by melatonin secretion, which exerts a suppressive effect on prolactin. Altered photoperiod (16:8 h light : dark) influences milk production in dairy cattle, but evidence for this relationship in sheep is scarce. The effect is mediated by greater circulating concentrations of IGF-I caused by long daily photoperiods, which in turn induces the mammary gland to increase milk production. Exposing the dairy cattle kept at high latitudes in winter sason to dim illumination at night and a minimum photoperiod of 12 h of light increase milk production.

Melatonin participates in the circadian GH-IGF-I axis activity. Melatonin might affect milk production as low melatonin level increase production of IGF-I in liver. This has been proved by melatonin administration to mimic a short-day photoperiod which suppresses increase in IGF-I in heifers induced by long days. Administration of melatonin in cows does not affect milk production but decrease milk production in sheep. Following injection, the melatonin concentration in milk increased rapidly and corresponds to serum value 15-30 minute later. However, more studies in cows and buffaloes needs to be carried out to clearly elicit the intractions of melatonin and serotonin in relation to prolactin and milk secretion.

❑❑❑

Chapter-24

Synthesis of Milk

Synthesis of milk constitutent takes place in the epithelial cells of mammary gland. Some of the constituents are being taken directly from the blood.

Milk fat synthesis

Fat content of milk varies considerably among species and the degree of unsaturation of long chain fatty acids of milk (TAG) differ among species. The synthesis of milk fat takes place in the cytoplasm of the epithelial cells. Milk fat of nonruminant contains higher proptotions of medium chain fatty acids (C8-C12), while elephant milk fat contain almost entirely medium chain fatty acids. Rabbit milk fat contains about 70 % of C8-C10 fatty acids. Milk fat of rat, mouse, human, monkey and ruminants contain notable proportions of these fatty acids. Medium chain fatty acids are synthesized denovo within the mammary gland and are incorporated directly into the milk tryaclyglycerol (TAG). These fatty acids are neither desaturated nor elongated into longer chain fatty acids. Milk fat also contain about 5-7 % short chain fatty acids (C4-C6) which are mainly contributed by BHBA.

Mammary gland easily synthesizes TAG with low melting point so that it can be easily secreted into milk as liquid droplets. The melting point of milk fat is lowered due to the following reasons.

1. Increased proportion of short and medium chain fatty acids
2. Asymmetric positioning of shorter chain fatty acids on glycerol backbone of the TAG.
3. Increased degree of unsaturation of long chain fatty acids.

In the bovine milk, 50 % of the milk fat is of denovo synthesis origin and the remaining is contributed either by dietary source or rumen lipid biosynthesis. Thus origin of the fat in the milk could be;

- *From the glycolysis of glucose.* The acetyl Co-A generated through pyruvate is the major source of fat synthesis in non-ruminants but ruminant cannot utilize this acetyl Co-A.
- *The dietary triacylglycerols.* The rumen synthesized triacylgycerols constitute second source of milk fat. These are absorbed from the GI wall and reaches to mammary gland in the form of low density lipoproteins through blood. The lipoprotein lipase enzyme in the wall of epithelial cell or capillary wall degrades them into fatty acids (C14, C16, C18), monoglycerides and glycerol which subsequently enter mammry cell for the milk fat synthesis. Only chylomicrons and low density fraction of plasma lipoprotein (1.005 to 1.010 dalton) contribute to TAG synthesis. Non-esterified fatty acids are present in low concentrations in the blood and AV difference is small. However there is a uptake and release of NEFA by the mammary gland.
- The third important source of milk fat is *de novo synthesis*. Mammary gland uses beta- hydroxyl butyric acid (BHBA) and acetate for local synthesis of fat. BHBA contribute to the first 4 carbon atom of the most of fatty acids synthesized by the mammary gland. Acetate contributes to C4-16 portions of the fatty acid.

Ruminant has glucose sparing mechanism for lactose production and utilization. This is achived by i) utilization of propionate for glucose production ii) Utilization of acetate for fat and energy purpose and iii) Absence of citrate cleavage pathway in adipose and mammary tissue of gland which prevent utilization of glucose for fat synthesis. In neonate calf the rumen fermentation is delayed so that glucose in lactose could be utilized and degradation of lactose in the rumen is delayed.

De novo synthesis of fat

In the ruminant, the carbon sources used for FA synthesis are acetate (the most important one) and β-hydroxybutyrate (BHBA). Glucose is a carbon source for FA synthesis in nonruminants. The reducing equivalents needed for FA synthesis come from NADPH2 (nicotinamide adenine dinucleotide phosphate, reduced form). The two key enzymes involved in fatty acid synthesis in the mammary gland are:

i) **Acetyl-CoA Carboxylase -** It is the rate limiting enzyme for the fatty acid synthesis pathway.

ii) **Fatty Acid Synthetase -** It is a large complex of enzyme activities responsible for the chain elongation of the fatty acid chains.

The relative proportions of milk fatty acids either from de novo synthesis or blood lipids are dependent on carbon chain length of the fatty acid. Short chain fatty acids arise predominantly from de novo synthesis in the epithelial cell, while longer chain fatty acids arise directly from blood lipids. An example is given in the table below for the cow milk.

Proportional contribution of sources of fatty acids in cow milk

Fatty Acid	% of FA from De novo synthesis	% of FA from VLDL Fatty Acid
C4 -C10	100	0
C12	80-90	10-20
C14	30-40	60-70
C16	20-30	70-80
C18	0	100

De novo synthesis of fat involves acetyl CoA as a main primer of malonyl CoA in the presence of enzyme Acetyl CoA carboxylase and ATP as energy source. There is a stepwise addition of 2-carbon chain of primer by fatty acid synthetase enzyme and nicotin adenine dinucleotide (NADH) reduction step in fatty acid synthesis. The fatty acid chain gradually increases in presence of different enzyme and the end product of synthesis is palmitic acid (C16.0). Later is released by action of long chain acylthioesterase (thioesterase I) component of enzyme from the FA synthetase enzyme complex. The medium chain acylthioesterase enzyme having molecular weight of 29000 (Thioesterase II) stops the lengthening of fatty acid chain at 8 or 10 carbon atom leading to release of medium chain fatty acids and its esterification into TAG. In the absence of this enzyme the elongation of fatty acid synthetase continues until chain length of 16 C atom (palmitic acid) is attained.

As per biohydrogenation theory milk fat depression (MFD) is caused by an inhibition of milk fat synthesis by specific fatty acids (FAs) which are produced as intermediates in ruminal biohydrogenation. The intermediates *Trans-10, cis-12 CLA isomers* inhibits milk fatty acid synthesis in a dose depend manner. Regulation by CLA occurs naturally in dairy cows when specific CLA isomers are produced in rumen biohydrogenation. This is a physiological example of nutritional genomics that is referred as diet-induced milk fat depression, It involves coordinated down-regulation of mRNA expression of key lipogenic enzymes like sterol response element-binding protein 1 (SREBP1), SREBP-activation proteins and Spot 14. The key lipogenic enzymes are transcriptionally regulated via SREBP1. SREBP1c and Spot 14 knock-out mice exhibit reduced milk fat similar to the magnitude and pattern of MFD in the cow.

$$\text{Acetyl CoA} + Co_2 + \text{ATP} \xrightarrow{\text{Acetyl CoA carboxylase}} \text{Malonyl CoA} + \text{ADP} + \text{Pi}$$

$$\text{Malonyl CoA} + \text{ACP} \underset{}{\overset{\text{Malonyl CoA -ACP transference}}{\rightleftarrows}} \text{Malonyl - ACP} + \text{CoA}$$

$$\text{Acetyl ACP} + \text{Malonyl ACP} \overset{\beta\text{- Ketoacyl synthetase}}{\rightleftarrows} \text{Acetoacetyl - ACP} + Co_2 + \text{ACP}$$

$$\text{Acetoacetyl - ACP} + \text{NADPH} \overset{\beta\text{- Ketoacyl reductase}}{\rightleftarrows} \text{D - }\beta\text{ - OH - butyrl ACP} + \text{NADP}$$

$$\text{D - }\beta\text{ - OH - butyrl - ACP} + \text{ACP} \overset{\beta\text{- hydroxyacyl dehydrogenase}}{\rightleftarrows} \text{Crotonyl - ACP} + H_2o$$

$$\text{Crotonyl – Acyl- ACP} + H_2o \overset{\text{Fatty Acid deacylase}}{\rightleftarrows} \text{Fatty Acid} + \text{ACP}$$

Fatty Acid Synthesis

Lactose synthesis

Lactose is the major sugar of milk and is synthesized in membrane of Golgi apparatus. Milk also contains little amounts of glycopeptides, glycoprotein, galactose, free glucose, oligosaccharides and nucleotide sugars. Lactose is made up of one molecule of glucose and galactose which join together at 1-4 C linkage. Lactose concentrations vary in different species and it maintains >50 % osmalality of milk. The brief pathway of synthesis of lacrtose is given below.

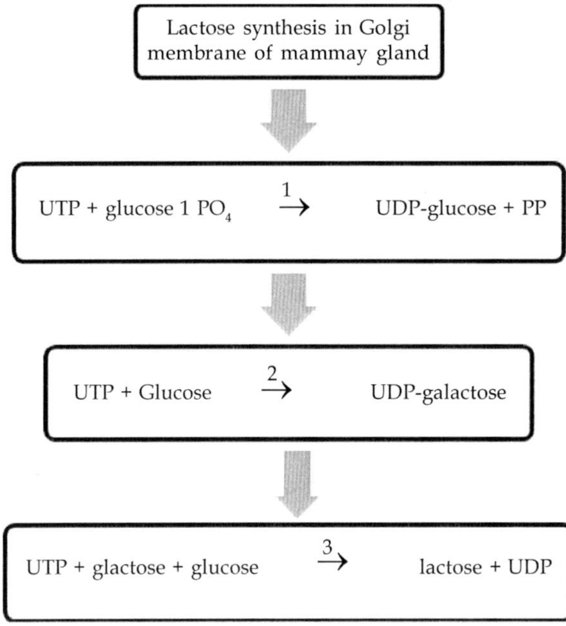

In lactose synthesis pathway the enzymes involed at step 1, 2, 3 are;

1. UDP glucose pryorphosphorylase
2. UDP glactose -4- epimerasecauses inversion of OH group on 4 C of UDP - glucose.
3. Lactose synthetase enzyme is an allosteriac enzyme. It consists of a two subnits i) α-lactalbumin and ii) β-galactosyltransferease (GT) enzyme. α-lactalbumin is present on the inner surface of golgi vesticles while galactosyltransferase is synthesized in RER and moves to golgi vesicles. The enzyme α-lactalbumin is also secreted into milk. Galactosyltransferease is present in the mammary gland and other tissue of body. This enzyme transfers UDP-glucsose to N-acetylglucosamine in body tissues. But in the mammary gland tissue, without α-lactalbumin, galactosyltransferase enzyme cannot synthesize lactose. α-lactalbumin catalyzes the attachment of galactose to *N*-acetylglucosamine units on glycoproteins. The presence of α-lactalbumin thus changes the specificity of galactosyltransferase enzyme so that it can transfer galactose to glucose. Although GT is found in many tissues in the body, alpha-lactalbumin is only found on the inner surface of the Golgi in the mammary glands. The mammary gland of goat and cows has been shown to absorb glucose from the blood stream during lactation. It

has been shown that lactose is formed when slices or suspensions of the mammary glands of guinea pig and rat are incubated with glucose. The enzyme galactosyltransferase transfers the UDP-glucsose to N-acetylglucosamine in body tissues in the way depticted below.

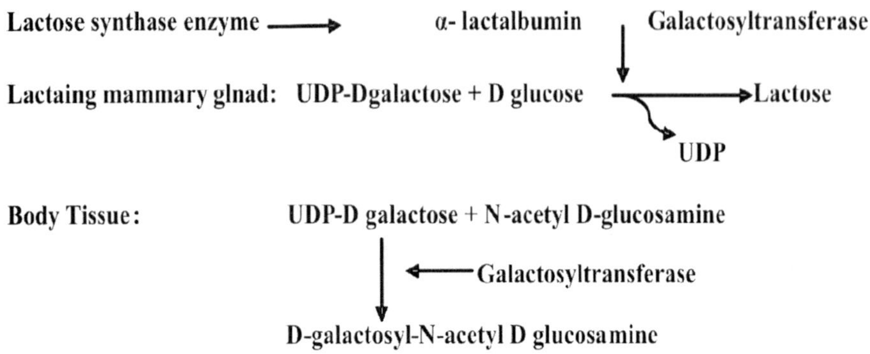

Role of galactosyltransferase enzyme in mammary gland and body tissues

Chapter-25

Somatic Cell Count of Milk

Introduction

Somatic cells are mainly milk-secreting epithelial cells that have been shed from the lining of the gland and WBC (leukocytes), that have entered the mammary gland in response to injury or infection. Somatic cells for milk include: 75% leukocytes (neutrophils, macrophages, lymphocytes) and 25% epithelial cells. Erythrocytes can also be found at the concentrations ranging from 0 to $1.51 x 10^6$ per ml.

In case of mastitis, the ratio just becomes reverse i.e., 25% leukocytes and 75% epithelial cells are found in milk. The leukocytes can even go upto 90% in severe mastitis. SCC > 100,000 cells/ml is considered as threshold for the California mastitis test (CMT) in dairy cows in India. Poor hygiene has been demonstrated to be associated with higher SCC and the risk of subclinical mastitis in dairy cattle. Higher SCC involves greater risk of raw milk contamination with pathogens and antibiotic residues. Normally, SCC is $< 1 x 10^5$ cells/ml in milk from a healthy mammary gland, while bacterial infection lead to $>1 x 10^6$ cells/ml.

Table. Somatic cells in different lacteal secretions

Type of mammary secretion	Milk somatic cells (%)			
	PMNL	Macrophages	Lymphocytes	Epithelial cells
Milk	3	80	16	2
Colostrum	62	35	4	0
Secretions at drying off	3	89	7	1

Milk Somatic cell counts

Factors that increase milk SCC	Factors that decrerase milk SCC
• Infection/injury of udder • Older animals • Newly calved animals • Extreme climate stress • Changing feeds • Mastitis • In-house overcrowding	• Better shelter hygiene and udder health • Complete milking of animal • Use of post milking teat dip with iodophore solutions • Effective mastitis management (CMT) • Feeding of vitamin E, Zn

Monitor the somatic cell counts of milk at monthly interval to avoid mastitis incidence and maintain the quality of milk.

Figure. Factors that affects somatic cell counts of milk in dairy animals

Effect of different factors on milk SCC

Factors such as parity, breed, stage of lactation, type of birth, monthly, seasonal variations and hygiene influence SCC of milk and may explain 48% of SCC variance. The SCC number is low in early lactation due to increase in milk yield and increase with decrease of milk yield in late lactation in different breeds of cows (Table). SCC number is significantly influenced by stages of lactation in Sahiwal and Karan fries cows.

Table. Breedwise somatic cell counts (x10^5 cells/ml) and milk yield (kg) during different stages of lactation

Days of	Tharparkar		Sahiwal		Karan Swiss		Karan Fries	
Lactation	SCC	MY	SCC	MY	SCC	MY	SCC	MY
01-30	1.26±0.18	6.12±0.28	1.20±0.08	8.50±0.76	1.71±0.32	6.12±0.18	1.63±0.08	11.12±0.62
31-60	1.47±0.37	8.25±0.65	1.33±0.14	9.37±1.19	1.67±0.24	7.96±0.99	1.40±0.10	15.46±4.20
61-90	1.05±0.05	7.70±0.56	1.12±0.06	9.50±0.64	1.76±0.25	8.27±0.67	1.72±0.09	10.47±0.87
91-120	1.29±0.11	6.59±0.70	1.28±0.08	7.06±0.54	1.35±0.19	9.84±1.19	1.67±0.12	10.59±0.69
121-150	1.74±0.84	6.25±1.25	1.61±0.18	7.64±0.53	2.03±0.34	8.25±1.01	1.69±0.13	9.98±0.66
151-180	1.50±0.27	6.00±0.65	1.39±0.19	8.61±0.59	1.82±0.33	7.85±0.56	1.73±0.14	9.52±0.67
181-210	1.36±0.23	5.00±0.81	1.54±0.24	7.12±0.47	1.28±0.25	8.62±1.47	1.64±0.12	8.25±0.54
211-240	1.04±0.16	4.16±0.33	1.80±0.44	6.50±0.64	1.39±0.17	6.95±1.05	1.81±0.14	8.13±0.47
241-270	1.20±0.17	4.62±0.71	1.32±0.21	6.00±0.50	1.12±0.04	6.00±1.38	1.39±0.07	8.48±0.42
271-300	1.12±0.22	2.85±0.49	1.25±0.19	3.33±0.88	1.33±0.20	8.21±1.10	1.37±0.72	9.12±0.62
301&Above	1.09±0.09	6.33±0.60	1.11±0.08	6.34±0.77	1.20±0.13	7.42±0.60	1.64±0.16	8.18±0.64
Overall Av.	1.26±0.06	5.95±0.31	1.31±0.04	7.90±0.26	1.54±0.07	7.85±0.29	1.61±0.03	10.17±0.43
Level of Significance	NS	NS	NS	**	NS	NS	NS	*

NS = Not sugbufucabtm * p<0.05, ** p<0.01; MY = milk yield, SCC = somatic cell count.

In goats, evening milking has higher SCC (17-78%) in milk than that obtained from the morning. However, buffaloes milked twice a day at regular intervals did not exhibit variation in milk SCC. Goats with multiple births have higher SCC than those of single birth. In buffalo milk, SCC was low during cold and hot dry season but were high in hot humid season, the values being 76000/ml, 1,08000/ml & 1,35000/ml, respectively. Long milking intervals with automatic milking systems (AMS) increase bulk milk SCC. Dairy ewes with pendulous udder had a higher SCC. Older animal's milk has higher SCC as compared to younger ones. Mean normal SCC values in milk of Indigenous Sahiwal and Tharparkar cows and the buffaloes are less than the crossbred dairy cows. Nutritional supplementation with vitamins and minerals enhances the immunity of the animal and therefore decreases SCC of milk. Cows can easily be checked for subclinical mastitis by the California Mastitis Test (CMT) at fortnightly intervals. This ensures control on incidence of mastitis and good udder halth is maintained. Relation between CMT and SCC of individual cows is shown in the table.

Average milk SCC in different breeds

Breed	SCC ($\times 10^5$ cells/ml)
Murrah	1.00
Tharparkar	1.26
Sahiwal	1.31
Karan Fries	1.61
Karan Swiss	1.54

CMT Score	Average Somatic Cell Count in Milk
Negative (no mastitis)	100,000
Trace (of mastitis)	300,000
Class 1 (light mastitis)	900,000
Class 2 (severe mastitis)	2,700,000
Class 3 (very severe mastitis)	8,100,000

Clean milk

Clean milk is defined as the raw milk obtained from healthy animals that has been produced and handled under hygienic conditions. Clean milk has a normal composition, possesses a natural milk flavour, contains least number of harmless bacteria but does not contain any hazardous chemical residues.

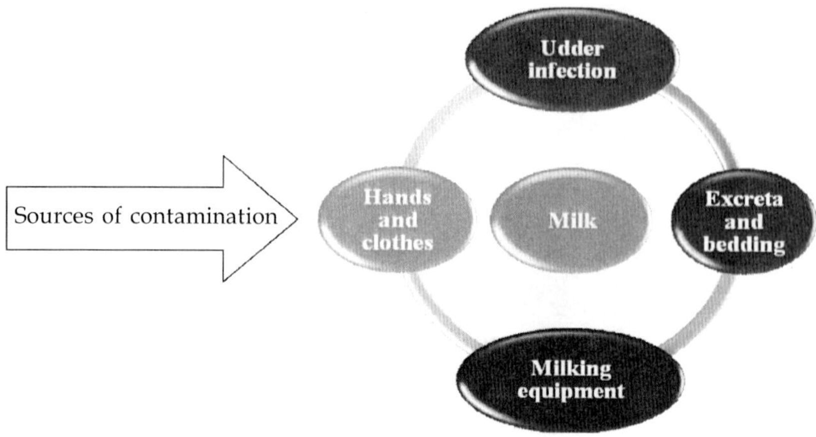

Figure. Relationship of Hygiene, Mastitis and SCC

Hygiene of dairy cows provides information about animal welfare and farm facilities. Numerous studies have indicated that effective implementation of best management practices results in reduced prevalence of IMI and reduced BTSCC. Lack of hygiene facilities and use of pond and lake water for drinking increases milk SCC. The method of udder cleaning also influence milk SCC as shown in the table.

Table. Effect of premilking udder-cleaning method on SCC.

Method of udder cleaning before milking	Mean (×1,000 cells/ml)
No contact with udder or wash only when dirty, n = 9	31.25
Dry wipe only, n = 39	215.35
Dry wipe and additional washing, n = 7	169.40
Wet wipe, n = 18	200.79
Washing with water, n = 2	265.67

Somatic cell counts can used as a proxy for subclinical mastitis detection with av. SCC>200,000 cells/ml. Cows with post-milking standing times of >90 minute have tendancy to have higher SCC. The Higher SCC in milk are often associated with more pendulous udders (9.6% increase in SCC/cm^2) and greater total cross-sectional area of the teats (7.2% increase in SCC/cm^2) in ewes. In a large herd use of composite milk samples overlook some subclinical infections cases due to dilution with milk from healthy quarters that contain few somatic cell counts.

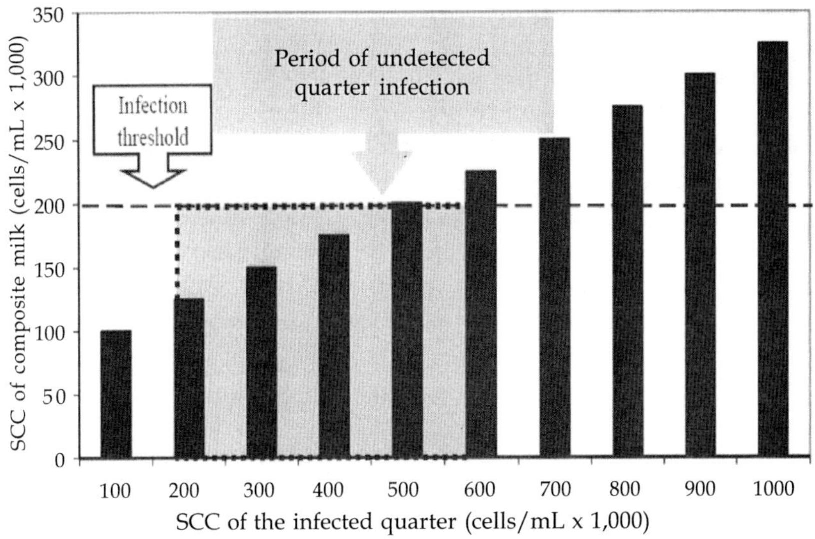

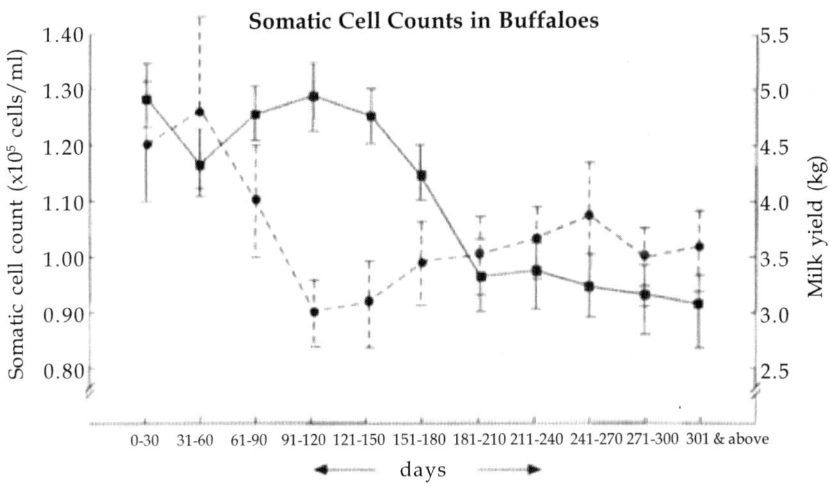

Figure. Somatic cell count (● ······· ●) and milk yield (■——■) during different stages of lactation in buffaloes

SCC standards

SCC limit is the key component of national and international regulation for milk quality. In US a standard of 750,000 cells/ml is preferred (National Conference on Interstate Milk Shipments, 2011). However, US processors seek to get milk at or below 250,000 cells/ml to maintain product shelf life and flavour. National standards for BTSCC vary from <400,000 cells/mL (EU, Australia, New Zealand and Canada) to <1,000,000 cells/mL (Brazil)).

Effect of SCC on milk components

The increase in milk SCC also influences milk quality and composition. SCC of individual cow's milk is significantly correlated with a decrease in milk constituents. Mastitis milk has higher SCC and low milk lactose, α-lactalbumin and fat in buffaloes. High SCC affects the yield of milk protein concentration and reduces the shelf life of pasteurized liquid milk. High SCC increases whey protein and decreases casein concentration which results in lesser cheese yields. Thus regular monitoring of individual cow SCC in a herd is an important tool that can be used by dairy farmers to get good quality milk. Proper milking techniques, improved sanitation, use of teat dip solutions and dry period management can maintain the SCC to normal level in a dairy farm. Appropriate climatic stress amelioration meaure should be used to give comfort to the cows and buffaloes to maintain normal somatic cell secretion in milk. SCC increase with increase in temperature and humidity during summer and decrease at low temperature in winter season. Increase in SCC have been reported to reduce the milk yield. Farmers need to be given incentives to produce milk with low SCC. At the same time dairy industry also needs to check the milk quality at receiving end with SCC index.

Table. Effect of season on milk SCC in different breeds (x10^5 cells/ml).

Season	Tharparkar	Sahiwal	Karan Swiss	Karan Fries	Buffalo
Winter	1.04 (0.86-1.26)	1.06 (0.75-1.39)	1.10 (0.71-1.62)	1.15 (0.77-1.77)	1.08 (0.27-2.46)
Hot humid	1.49 (0.90-2.58)	1.61 (0.73-2.59)	2.46 (0.91-3.92)	2.28 (0.71-3.92)	1.36 (0.35-3.86)
Hot dry	1.10 (0.56-2.55)	1.12 (0.56-2.15)	0.98 (0.60-2.20)	1.11 (0.56-3.88)	0.76 (0.40-1.22)

Table. Effect of somatic cell count on milk production.

SSCx10^5 cells/ml	Decrease in milk yield/cow/day
50,000	0.0
100,000	0.7
200,000	1.4
400,000	2.0
800,000	2.7
1,600,000	3.4

❑❑❑

Chapter-26

Clean Milk Production and Milking Management

Milk is one of the important natural secretions from the mammary gland. It contains fat, protein, lactose, vitamins, minerals and large quantity of water to meet energy and other requirements of the body. These nutrients are present in a very easily digestible form so that even a neonate calf or human child could digest easily. Therefore, milk has been called as *Balance Food*. World trade organization (WTO) has recommended certain guidelines to strictly monitor the quality of milk. Indian farmers have to compete with the global market for value addition of milk and milk product export. This could be achieved only when clean and hygiene milk production practices are followed by the dairy farmers in field and farm conditions. In our country, total number of lactating animals is 90 millions which are being maintained by 90 million rural populations. This indicates that one animal is being maintained by each person/farmer. Therefore contribution of the farmers in clean milk production is immense. Clean milk production implies to cleanliness of the shelter, hygienic milking and feeding practices and above all, a sound udder health of animal.

What is milk?

Milk is an opaque white liquid produced by the mammary gland of mammals. It provides the primary source of nutrition for young mammals before they are able to digest other types of food.

What is clean milk?

Clean milk can be defined as the fresh milk which have normal composition and is free from any foreign particles (dust, hairs, bacteria etc.) and drugs residues. There can be adverse effect on its quality if proper care is not taken during production, procurement and transport. The quality of milk products like ghee, powder, butter, paneer, curd, buttermilk, sweets etc. depends on process and quality of raw material. If raw milk has good quality, then finished product will have better shelf life. Clean milk can be obtained from a healthy animal by following the hygienic milking management practices. Incidence of mastitis impair milk synthesis and the quality of milk.

Mastitis

Mastitis is a disease which occurs due to infection in secretory tissue of mammary gland. It can be easily characterized by symptoms like warmness/ redness of udder, fever, difficult milking, watery milk, yellowish milk, flakes and pus in milk, blood clots or pinkish milk and a swollen udder. Mastitis may occur due to unhygienic milking practices, spoiled feed intake, unhygienic floor of shelter and is caused by bacterial infection (Figure). Mastitis decreases milk yield and alter milk composition (Table). Mastitis can be diagnosed by palpation of inflamed udder by hand and change in milk composition. If animal exhibit pain in udder and is restless, it indicates infection in the udder. Different stages of mastitis could be charactersied by the symptoms as given in Table.

- Buffaloes suffer less from mastitis than the cows due to tight teat sphincter muscle.
- High producing cows suffer more from mastitis than the low milk producers.
- Cull the cows with repeat mastitis history.

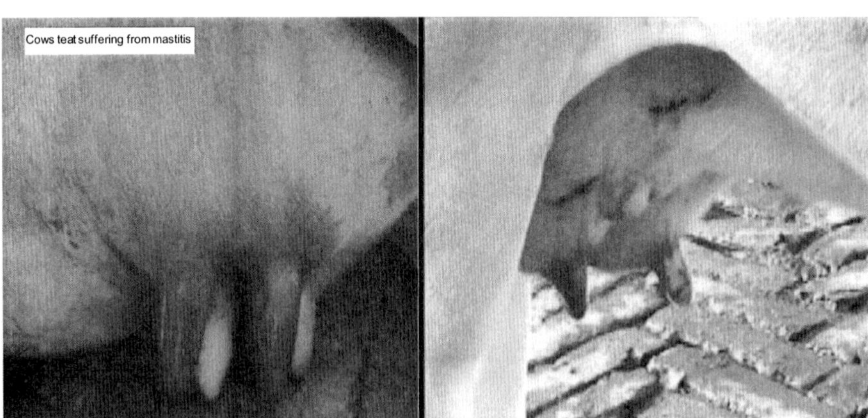

Figure. A blind teat and dead quarter of udder due to mastitis

Table. Milk yield and its compositional changes associated with mastitis.

Constituents	Cow milk		Buffalo milk	
	Normal	Mastitis	Normal	Mastitis
Milk yield (kg)	18.73	0.36	8.06	0.49
Fat (%)	4.54	2.46	7.26	3.46
Protein (%)	2.96	3.53	4.89	6.02
Lactose (%)	4.69	3.62	4.51	3.66
pH	6.47	7.16	6.48	7.16
Electrical conductivity (mhos)	2.31	3.71	2.56	3.53
NEFA (mM/l)	0.15	0.08	0.16	0.08
Chloride (mg %)	108.25	165.48	92.12	163.97

Table. Different stages of mastitis incidence.

Stages of mastitis	Symptoms
1. Chronic stage	No-visible sign
2. Sub-acute or sub-clinical stage	Slight changes in milk composition, bacteria appears in milk, no systemic visible sign
3. Clinical/Acute stage - Mild - Severe	Appearance of flakes, clots, swelling of udder, fever, loss of appetite, deprenia, weakness, rapid pulse , dehydration, hot quarter, rise in body temperature
4. Per-acute stage	Animal exhibit severe symptoms (as above) followed by death of animal

Precautions for checking the incidence of mastitis

- Shelter of the animals should be well ventilated for effective dryness of floor to avoid animal injury/ lameness.
- All feeding stalls and floor/beds should be kept clean dry.
- Regular spray of lime at monthly intervals should be done on floor to check growth of pathogens.
- Lactating animals should be fed vitamin E (@ 1g/ d) with concentrate mixture to improve udder health, milk quality and to reduce mastitis incidence.
- The milking area should be kept clean and dry.

  It should have a

  - Clean water supply facilities;

- Have waste handling facilities;
- Have well ventilation/ fan availability for comfort at milking during summer
- Animal excreta should be disposed off away from milking area.

- Farmers should ensure hand or machine milking is carried out under hygienic conditions
- Wash the udder and teat of animals with iodine solution or savalon before milking so that dirt, hairs, dusts particles etc. does not pass into the milk.
- Healthy animals should be milked first. Animals suffering from mastitis should be milked afterwards to avoid contamination of normal milk with mastitis milk.
- Discard/ dispose off mastitis milk away from the animal shelter.
- Check the quality of milk. The first step is fore- strip each teat three times. Examine the milk quality for any abnormal milk colour and consistacny.
- Dry the teat and teat ends with individual cloth piece/towel. Cleanliness of teat and udder reduces incidence of clinical mastitis and improves milk quality.
- Teats may be dipped in a disinfectant solution (savalon/potassium permanganate or iodine solution) after the milking to maintain udder health.
- After completion of milking, teat pore of animal remain open for about 30 minutes. Bacteria may enter into the mammary gland through opened teat pore if animal sits on ground after milking. Offering of fodder after milking engage the cow in ingesting the food and prevent entry of bacteria in teats.
- Check milk pH and use mastitis strips for detection of mastitis at least at 15 day intervals.

Table. Factors that influences letdown of milk in cows and buffaloes

Factors that stimualte letdown of milk	Factors that reduce or inhibit letdown of milk
Sight of calves, time of milking	Stress –climatic, fever
Sight of milking place	Sickness, diseases
Sight of *Milker* (men/women)	Abnormal/delayed parturition
Sight of concentrate feed/fodder	Dystocia
Washing of udder	Retention of fetal membranes
Washing of teat, sound of milking pails	Abnormal sounds, thunder storms, barking of dogs, cat presence at the time of milking
Calf suckling	Beating of animal at milking
Teat and udder message	Stranger/large noises
Congenial/silent milking environment	Death of calf

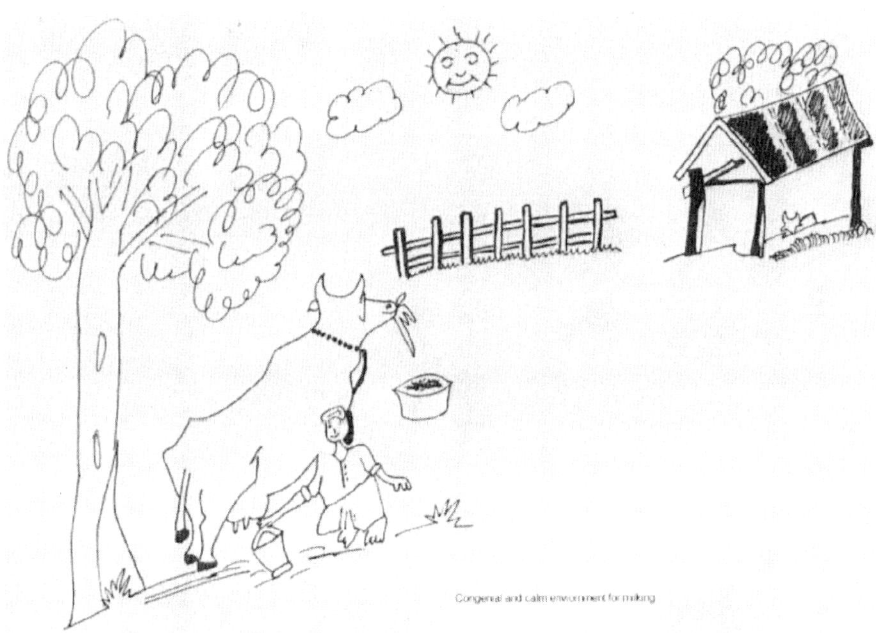

Figure. Congenial environment for complete milking.

Mechanism of Milk let down

Let-down of milk in cows and buffaloes are initialed by hand or milking stimulus such as suckling by calf (Figure). The sensory signals are transmitted from teat to the hypothalamus (brain) and release intrinsic (normal) oxytocin from the posterior pituitary gland. Oxytocin reaches to mammary gland through blood and binds with myoepithelial cells. These cells contracts and release milk in the lumen of alveoli. Thus, milk which is stored in alveoli passes into lower part of udder due to milking or hand stimulus. This mechanism is known as *Neuro-endocrine reflex* and has been depicted. For complete let-down of milk, teat and udder message should be done fully so that all the milk is taken out during milking. Partial letdown of milk reduces milk yield and less fat. The half life of oxytocin is only 2 minutes in blood circulation and it vanishes from blood within 2-5 minutes. Thus milking should be completed within 5-6 minutes as milk flow is maximum during this period of time.

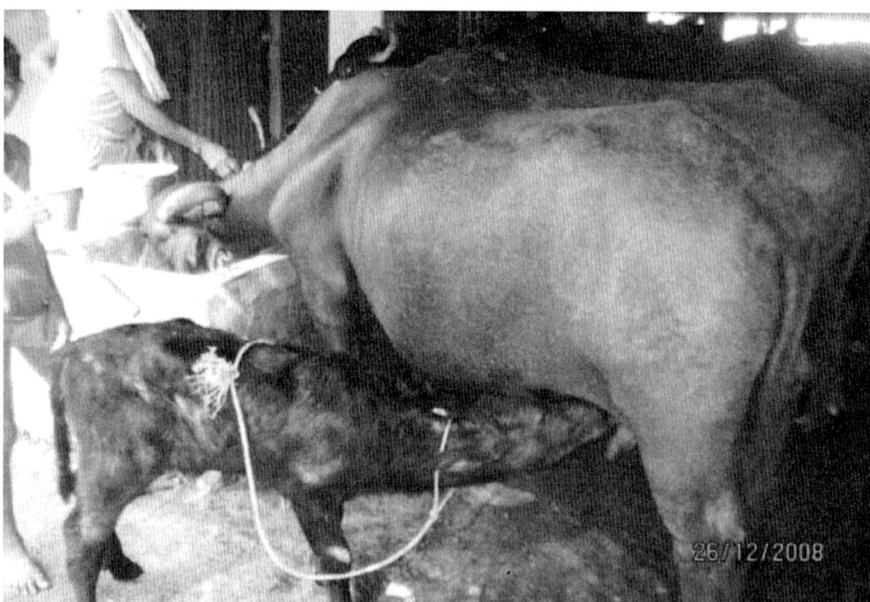

Figure 8. Let down of milk by calf suckling

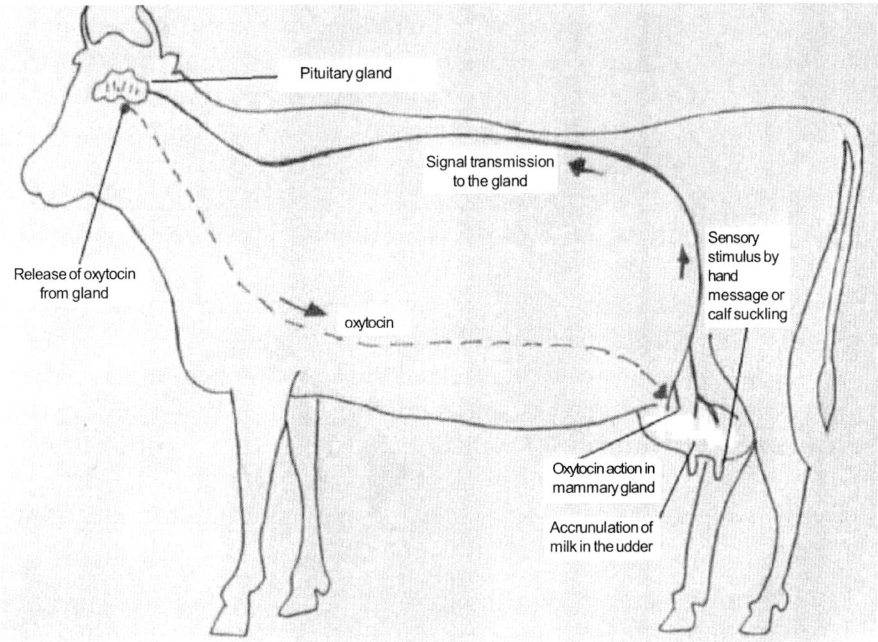

Figure. The process of let-down of milk in a cow (Neuro-edocrine reflex)

Role of oxytocin in maternal behavoir and Bonding

It has been postulated that oxytocin (OT) and Vasopressin (VP) have distinct but opposing functions. Vasopressin play a role in homeostatic regulation of body fluid, temperature, cardiovascular and autonomic nervous system functions. VP may lead to an increase in arousal, attention, and aggression through activation of these systems. OT is more involved in regulation of prosocial behaviors and may inhibit the actions of VP during pregnancy and lactation. Substantial animal research indicates role of OT in maternal behavior and bonding with neonate. An association between OT and maternal behavior has been found in rat, mice, heifer, pig and sheep. Rats receiving good maternal care and brief isolation in early infancy stage have higher OT receptor binding in brain areas than the one receiving longer isolation and less care. The specific areas of brain implicated in OT related functions are bed nucleus of stria terminalis, medial preoptic area and lateral septum. The higher OT levels during pregnancy facilitate postnatal maternal behavior and emotional bonding between mother and infant in humans. This bonding ensures safety and nurturing of a neonate in the beginning and establishes relationships later on. The *medial preoptic area* of brain has been identified as a major site for oxytocin and vasopressin-mediated maternal care. Further release of oxytocin and vasopressin and their receptor activation in central amygdala and bed nucleus of stria terminalis plays an important role for maternal aggression. During peri-parturient period there is an increased expression and intracerebral release of oxytocin and vasopressin in mammals. The onset of maternal behavior postpartum has also been attributed to decline in progesterone, increased estradiol and prolactin levels before parturition. But role of epinephrine, norepinephrine and serotonin still needs to be elucidated. The release of higher oxytocin level during after one hour of parturition is attenuated by factors like suckling, touching of breast and crying by a neonate in humans. Mothers possessing higher cortisol levels often have less caring and more aggressiveness towards their offspring. However, higher cortisol is associated with increased alertness of mother towards smell and sounds of a child.

Female rat having high anxiety- related behaviour (HAB) have four times more anxiety compared with low anxiety group (LAB) dams. The HAB dams display an intense and protective mothering style whereas LAB dams display only low maternal care due to oxytocin. Manipulation of brain oxytocin and vasopressin systems alters maternal behaviour, maternal aggression, maternal performance and dam's anxiety. Administration of oxytocin receptor antagonist into paraventricular nuclei reduces maternal aggression in HAB whereas oxytocin infusion increases aggression toward intruder in LAB dams. Vasopressin regulates important aspects of social behaviour in male and females. Brain vasopressin regulates fine-tuned maintenance of maternal care and maternal aggressive behaviour in lactating rat. Increased vasopressin release within the central amygdale and not in paraventricular nucleus in HAB than the LAB dams during maternal aggression.

Milking methods

Milking is the act of removing milk from the mammary gland. Milking of animal is done by hand or machine. Milking can be divided into following sub-tasks.

1. Collecting the animals before milking,
2. Routing the animals into the milking byre or milking place
3. Order of milking –

- Milk the high yielding animals
- Milk the healthy first calved animals
- Milk the adult animals free from mastitis
- Milk the cows which have mastitis or any other infection

4. Offer concentrate mixture and green fodder/ wheat straw
5. Inspection and cleaning of teats and udder
6. Teat message by hand/ or calf suckling to let-down milk
7. Fore- stripping and examination of milk quality
8. Milking by hand or machine
9. Removal of milking equipment and washing of udder
10. Routing the animals out of milking place

Generally, farmers milk the animals in the place of tying and no separate milking place is used. However, progressive dairy farms/ government dairy farms having more than 50 animals have separate milking place to milk the animals.

i) Method of hand milking

Most of the animals in small and medium dairy farms are milked by hand. A proper hygiene during hand milking is very essential. It is necessary that milkers should wash and dry their hand prior to milking. The place of milking should be cleaned before animal is being milked. Teats should be washed with clean water and dried. Hand milking is performed by messaging and pulling down of teat of the cow's udder and squirting the milk into a bucket by following methods.

a) **By fingers**: In this method milking is done by pressing of teat between the thumb and two forefingers. This result in trapping the milk in the lower part of teat, which is then squeezed out by the other fingers. This practice is good for animals which have small teats, but animals with large teat feel discomfort and teat injury may occur.

b) **Milking with full hand/ Fisting method :** In this method teat is grasped with a full-hand grip, and milking is done by use of all fingers and the palm (Figure). The upper end of the teat is closed off using the thumb and the forefinger. The teats are squeezed between the palm and the fingers forcing the milk out. This is the most accepted method of milking as it is similar to the calf suckling.

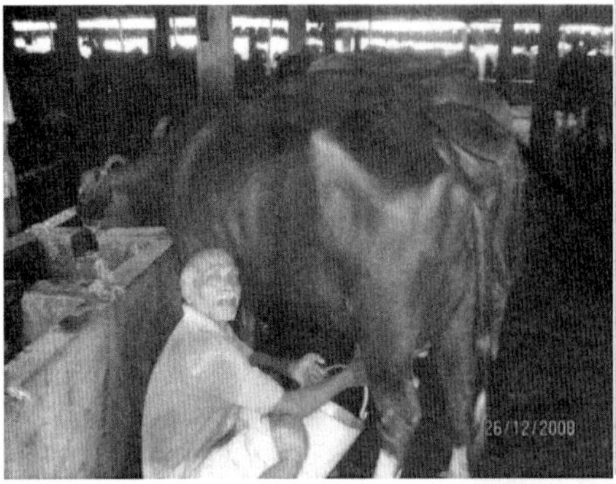

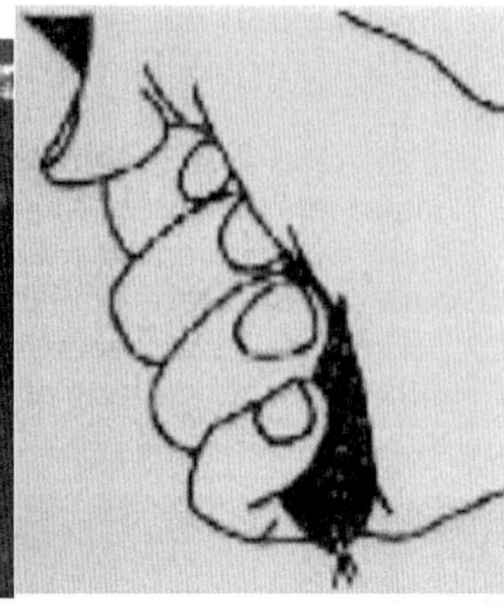

Figure. Hand Milking of a buffalo Full hand milking of a cow

ii) Machine milking operations

Progressive dairy farmers/large dairy farms and the organized herds generally use milking machine to milk the animals. Following two types of milking machine are commonly used to milk the animals.

a) **Bucket milking machines**: This is the most basic machine milking system for dairy animals. It can be used with stationary or portable units. Bucket milking machine is relatively cheap and is being used in small and large commercial farms. Animal are milked in tied conditions. Milk received in cans is recorded for its yields on a balance and carried manually.

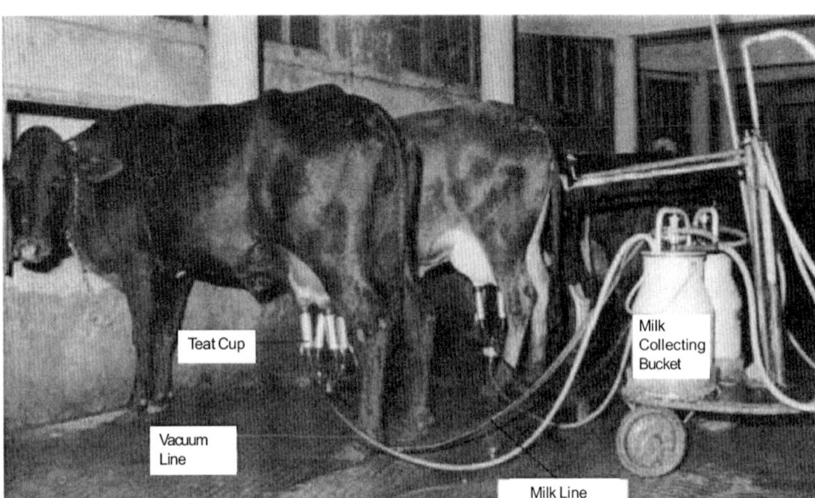

Figure. Bucket machine milking

c) **Pipeline milking system**: This type of milking system is popular method for milking large number of animals. The animals are machine milked in the stalls and milk is transported via a pipeline to the receiving unit where it is pumped into a cooling tank or milk containers. In this method animals milk yield is recoded manually. Now-a-days modern milking parlours like Vario tandem and Flat barn parlours, are available in which animal movement into milk parlour, milking, recording of milk yield, transport of milk into milk tank and washing of equipments are automatic and controlled through sensors tag fixed on animals body (Figure).

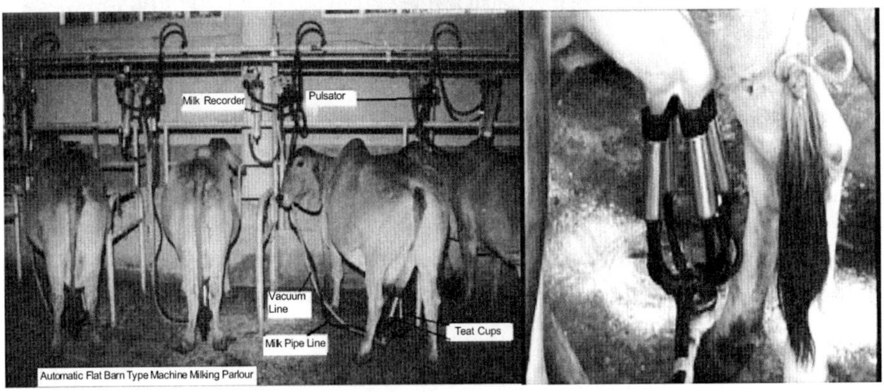

Figure. Sahiwal cows milked in a Flat Barn machine milking byre

Major components of machine milking

Vacuum supply unit- It has vacuum pumps and a gauge to show the pressure (mmHg).

Milking unit it has following components-

- Long milk tubes.
- A pulsator -which has a pulsation ratio of 50:50 or 40:60.
- Four teat cups innsulated with rubber liner.
- Clusters.
- A suction assembly unit and an air bubble free gasket milk bucket to receive the milk.
- A unit of transport and collection of milk.

Pressure gauze meter

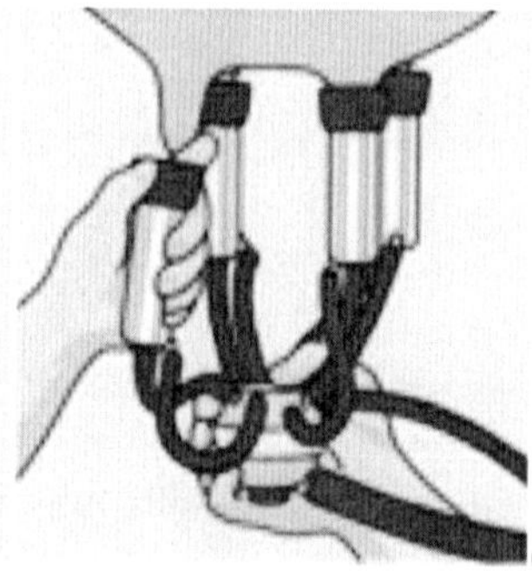

Application of teat cup

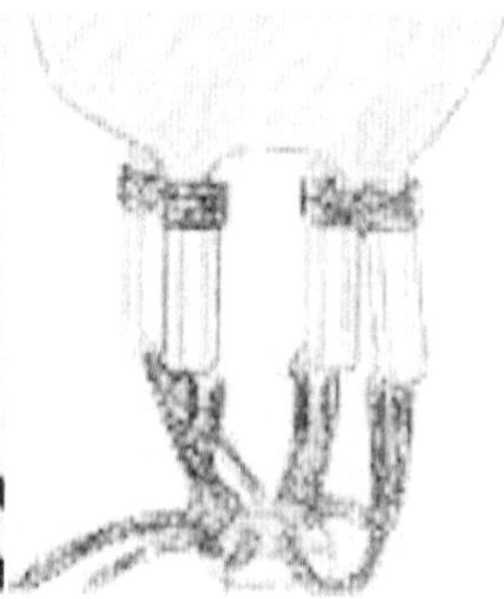

Teat cup attached to teat

Process of machine milking

In machine milking, *cups* are attached to all the four teats of a cow after cleaning the teat and udder (Figure). Vacuum pump creates a suction pressure to attatch teat cups while atmospheric air admitted into the pulsation chamber @once/seconds (the pulsation rate), allow the teat liner to collapse around the end of teat and relieve congestion in the teat tissue. Thus pulsator stimulates effective contraction and relaxation to the teat as being done by hand. The ratio of time that the liner is open (milking phase) and closed (rest phase) is called the *pulsation ratio.* The teat cups alternate between vacuum and normal air pressure to extract the milk without damaging teat of the cow.

The short milk tubes from teat cups brings the milk into the claw from where it passes through the long milk tubes into a milk line and then into the milk receiver. In bucket milking machine, milk directly goes into the milk bucket through tubes at the end of milking. The vacuum pump is allowed to remove the suction and teat cups are detached.

Advantages of machine milking

1. Machine is easily adaptable to cows and buffaloes.
2. It is easy to operate and cost economic. Machine milks 1.5 litre to 2 litres of milk/ minute.
3. Milk is very hygienic.
4. It ensures complete and efficient milking of animals
5. Machine milking save time.

Maintenance of milking machines

- Clean the different components of machine after each milking by recommended detergent.
- Clean dirt and other filth from the milk claw's air vents to speed up the milking process.
- Check rubber liners and discard the defective liners for better teat and udder health .
- Make sure that milk pipeline has the proper slant and that there are no leaks.
- Service the pump at intervals as per service manual.
- Maintain the oil level in the pump or supply cup and check the belt for proper alignment and tension.
- Clean valves, screen and filters. Make sure that air tubes, milk tube and liners are in good condition.
- Check and clean the controller at least at fortnightly intervals.
- Accumulation of dirt in the valve is one of the primary causes of malfunction.
- Clean the valves regularly.
- Check the pulsation ratio which may vary from 50:50 to about 70:30. Cows can be milked faster with a wider ratio. Longer milk phase and shorter rest phase may cause teat end trauma.

Chapter-27

Dairy Husbandry Practices for Clean Milk Production

There are simple check points that should be followed to produce quality milk from the animals.

Ensure milking under hygienic conditions

- Cleanliness of animals is a pre-requisite for the clean milk production. Animals soiled with dung, mud and ticks contaminate the milk.
- The place of milking should be dry and clean so that the animals are comfortable during the milking.
- Lactating Animals should be washed/ given water bath before milking at least once in winter months (morning) and twice during the summer month (morning and evening) to make them clean.
- In case of availability of separate milking parlours (place), animals should be given bath prior to milking.
- If separate space for milking is not available, then clean the floor before milking the animal.
- Wash the udder and teat of animals before milking so that dirt, hairs, dusts particles etc. does not pass into the milk during milking.
- Healthy animals should be milked first and the animals suffering from mastitis should be milked afterwards to avoid contamination of normal milk with mastitis milk.
- Don't mix mastitis milk with the normal milk. Discard/ dispose off mastitis milk away from the animal shelter.
- Check the quality of milk. The first step is forestrip each teat three times. Examine the milk quality. Fore- stripping is critical to the production of quality milk and fast milking times.

- Drying the teat and teat ends with individual cloth piece/towel is the most important step. Cleanliness of teat and udder reduces incidence of clinical mastitis and milk quality improves.
- Manual pre-stimulation of teats results in better let-down of milk and shorten milking time.
- Teats may be dipped in a disinfectant solution (Savlon, potassium permanganate or iodine solution) after the milking to maintain udder health.
- After the completion of milking, teat pores of animal remains open for about 25-30 minutes. Bacteria may enter into the mammary gland through opened teat pore if animal sits on ground after milking. Offering of fodder after milking engage the cow in ingesting the food and prevent entry of bacteria in teats.
- Check milk pH and use mastitis strips for detection of mastitis at intervals. If animal exhibit initial symptoms of pain and change in milk composition, feeding of citric acid (125 gm in water) helps in controlling the mastitis.
- Do not use oxytocin for let-down of milk. Farmers have misconception about oxytocin that it increases milk yield. The fact is that it does not increase milk production of cows and buffaloes.
- Filter the milk through a sieve or muslin cloth to remove undesirable foreign particles.

Ensure overall hygiene in the shelter

- Shelter of the animals should be well ventilated for effective dryness of floor and to avoid animal injury/lameness.
- All feeding stalls and floor/beds should be kept clean and dry.
- Sand bedding and fan can be used in summer to check decline in milk yield and quality.
- Regularly clean or scrape the passageways to remove animal excreta/dung.
- Regular spray of lime at monthly intervals should be done in animal houses to check growth of pathogens and disease incidence.

Ensure appropriate storage conditions

- Ensure that feed is protected from contaminants. Farmers should store and handle pesticides, treated seeds, medicated feed and fertilizers away from the milking area to avoid contamination of milk.
- Hay and dry feeds should be protected from a moist/humid environment.
- If silage is being used to feed the animals, it should be kept under sealed conditions.
- Avoid feeding of spoiled/mouldy stock feed to milking animals as these may contain poisonous fungal toxins/aflatoxins that can be transferred to milk.
- Feeding mangers should be cleaned, white washed with lime so that pathogens do not spoil the feed.
- Offer the feed/concentrate mixture at the time of milking based on milk production. Animal remains busy in taking the feed and gives milk without any trouble. At the same time complete milking can be done easily.
- Lactating animals should be fed vitamin E (@ 1g/d) with concentrate mixture to improve udder health and quality of milk.
- Always discard the residual feed/left over feeds.

Ensure clean water supply

A sufficient supply of clean water should be available for drinking, milking operations and for cleaning of equipments. Water is important constituents of milk in different breeds (Table). Restriction of water to lactating animals decease milk production.

Cleanliness of milk containers:

- Milk tanks/bucket/cans should be cleaned and dry to check growth of bacteria.
- Machine milking equipments should be regularly washed with detergents and dry in an open area after the milking.
- Use of warm water removes fat and protein residues effectively.

Steps in Clean Milk Production

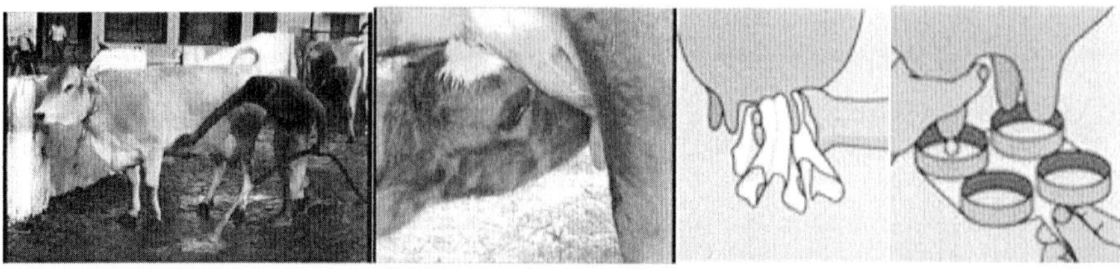

1. Wash the animals 2. Milk Let down by suckling 3. Clean the teats 4. Test milk by CMT

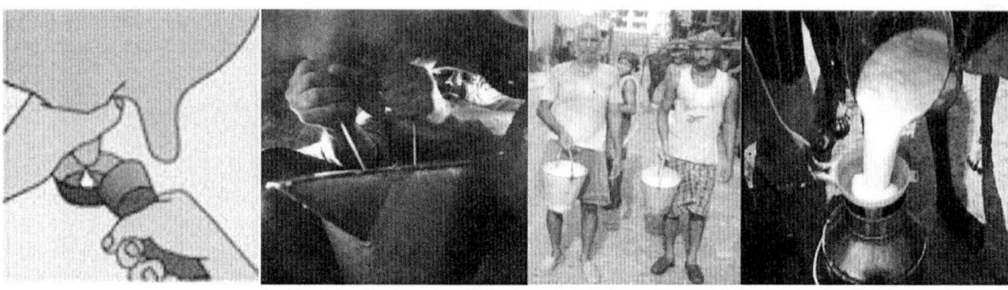

5. Observe quality of milk 6. Milk the animal 7. Pour the milk in container 8. Filter the milk

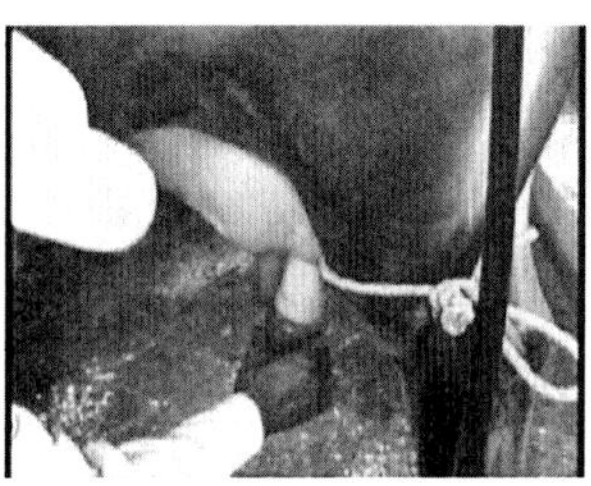

Application of teat dip solution after milking

Ensure milkers hygiene

Milker health may also affect quality and quantity of milk. Milker should be free from any infectious diseases like flu, cough, tuberculosis (TB) infectious disease. Pathogens of TB and brucella diseases may pass into milk or from man to animal and vice versa. Therefore, milker should take the following precautions.

- Keep hands and arms clean
- Should have trimmed nails to avoid injury to teat.
- Should not smoke during milking of animal
- Cover the mouth during sneeze or cough
- Wear suitable and clean working clothes
- Cover the head with turban/cloth to avoid falling of hairs into milk
- Cover the cuts or wounds if any, on body

Ensure milking routines

Milking routine is essential to maintain normal milk production and quality of milk.

- Milk the animal in a noise free area. Do not change the place of milking frequently.
- Always milk a clean, dry and well stimulated teat
- Milk the animals as per daily time schedule to ensure conditioned reflex.
- Ensure that animals are free from fear/ stress to express maximum milk yield potential during milking.
- Avoid rough milking practices as they may injure cows/ buffaloes udder health.
- Do not milk the animal very fast or slow. Milk the animal gently.
- Milk the cow completely. Incomplete milking or poor milking can affect cow well-being and milk production performance.
- Milking equipment should be well maintained and regularly serviced.

Ensure milk is handled properly after milking

- Milk hygiene and quality can only be maintained if care is taken in handling the milk. Milk should be stored in stainless steel containers solely used for this purpose.
- The lid of the container should fit tightly to prevent entry of dirt particles as well as entry of small insects, flies etc. into the container.
- Milk container should be handled with care and thoroughly washed after usage.
- Handle the milk gently. Milk is sensitive to stirring and shaking as this may damage the fat globules, leading to spoiled milk

Ensure milk quality

- In Organoleptic test simple normal senses of sight, smell and taste of milk is recorded to measure the overall quality. The result of test is obtained immediately on the spot.
- Cool the milk as soon as possible after milking to the required storage temperature (4-6 °C).

Table. Organoleptic test of milk

Parameters	Milk quality	Causes
A. Abnormal colour/ consistency	Pink Yellowish Blue thin color Large Clots or flakes Small white clots or grains Visible dirt and impurities	Blood contamination Colostrums or late milk Water adulterated Mastitis milk or sour milk Mastitis milk or adulterated with flour and skim milk powder. Unhygienic milking conditions
B. Abnormal smell and/or taste	Sour milk Blue souring Souring Malt Fruit aroma, Slimy milk, Bubbles, coagulation and whey separation	Lactose fermenting, acid producing bacteria Unpleasant sweet and sour smell, thin and waterish appearance caused by bacterial activity and storage in a closed container without ventilation *Streptococcus lactis var. maltigenes* Bitter: Peptonising of milk by *Streptococcus liquefraciens* Pseudomonas fragi producing esters Capsule forming bacteria, e.g. Aerobacter aerogenes and Alcaligenes viscosus Fermentation by yeast
C. Chemical changes	More Na and Cl and low lactose, Boiled Rancidity, Tallow	Mastitis milk, colostrums Release of volatile sulphides Lipolysis of fat Oxidation of fat
D. Off-flavors	Garlic, onion, beets, bad silage, certain plants and pastures	cause off-flavours to milk
E. Absorption of off-flavours from air, milk containers etc.	milk and cream	Absorb smelling compounds from the air. Strongly smelling paints, disinfectants and other chemicals should be not handled and stored in places where the dairy animals are kept and milked. Storage of milk together with fruits and fish also causes off-flavours to milk.

Preservation of milk at the farm

Storage of milk

Milk leaves the udder at approx. 35^{0}C and must be cooled quickly. Milk retains natural resistance to bacteria immediately after milking. The quality of milk may deteriorate if it is not handled under hygiene conditions after the milking. Proper cooling measures avoid bacterial growth and helps in maintaining the good flavours, color, high nutritive values and shelf life of milk. The quality of milk is generally relates to its chemical, microbiological and physical properties. Following points should be taken care for the safe storage of milk.

- Milk storage area should be clean and clear of accumulated rubbish, flies, dust and any chemical substances or unwanted materials which may be introduced into the feed, water or milk.
- Milk should be stored away from the milking area.
- Farmer should use separate room/site for storing the milk.
- Do not keep the milking cans in an open area/sunlight.

The chilled milk can be stored either in milk cans or in bulk milk cooling tanks. Bulk milk tank is a large storage tank for cooling and storage of milk at a cold temperature until it is transported to factory or milk plant. It consists of inner and outer tank sheets of high quality stainless steel. These tanks are used to store the raw milk on the farm in good condition.

Cooling

When raw milk is left standing for a while, it turns sour. Milk gets sour due to fermentation of lactose (milk sugar) into lactic acid by the bacteria. Rapid cooling of milk within 1-3hours at a temperature of 4-6°C prevents bacterial growth. At low temperature, chemical processes in milk are slowed down and milk spoilage is delayed. Thus cooling is the best means to maintain the freshness of the milk and to prevent bacteria from multiplying. Cooling practices depends on the milk quantity produced at the farm. Cooling does not necessary require expensive cooling equipment. Some simple and cheap methods are listed below. To obtain the best results with these methods, the container should be of metal (stainless steel or aluminum) for fast heat exchange.

- Shade and draught provide some cooling to the fresh milk. Covering the container with a wet cloth/gunny bags provides additional cooling from water evaporation. This method is practically useful in dry climates during the summer season.
- Air cooling is most effective at night. Evening milk could be stored without change of milk quality until next morning if the air temperature is <10°C.

Water cooling

Milk container can be put in the coldest or ice water available. It can also be kept in a metal basin or in earthen pit with running water, so that the water never warms up.

- A water stream could also be used to cool the milk as it functions equally well. For this type of cooling, the milk container should not be heavier.
- A slightly more sophisticated way of cooling with water is by having a double walls milk container. Milk is poured into the container and heat is exchanged with the water running in the double wall. This requires some kind of stirring and a large lid.
- For water cooling to be efficient, the temperature of water should be<20°C. It also requires a rich supply of clean water.

Ice cooling

Ice cooling is quite effective but expensive. Ice blocks can be put around the milk container. It is not advisable to put ice into the milk. Firstly the milk becomes diluted and, secondly, if water for ice making is not perfectly clean, it will add bacteria to the milk.

- If ice is readily available and not too expensive it can be combined with water cooling, which chill the water further.

Mechanical cooling

Mechanical cooling can be more or less expensive. If the farmer has a household refrigerator, this can be used for cooling the milk. How large a quantity of milk depends on the size of the refrigerator?

- Sophisticated coolers for chilling larger quantities of milk (Bulk milk tank) quickly are available from many agricultural companies.

Transporting the milk

High temperatures and long transportation times in unsanitary containers result in faster multiplication of bacteria in milk. Due to this large amount of the milk is spoiled before it reaches to milk processing plant. Transportation of milk should preferably be done in large containers/tankers as large quantity of milk heats up more slowly than small quantity.

- Increase in temperature during the transportation should be avoided as much as possible.
- If cooling of milk is impossible, preservatives can be used to retain milk quality until it reaches to dairy plant.
- A preservative (lactoperoxidase) preserve the milk and does not improve the quality of milk. It is a safe method of preserving milk if used correctly. It does not affect the quality of milk negatively.

Milking management of lactating animal is one of the important tasks in a dairy farm. To produce clean and quality milk, lactating animals should be healthy and be managed in an eco-friendly shelter and environment. Animals should be offered quality feed and fodder. In no case lactating animal should be given feed with foul smell or deteriorated fodder and feed. Animal can be milked with hand or machine. Clean, dry and well stimulated animals should be milked completely in a calm and comfortable environment. Milking operations should be hygienic and be carried out efficiently to get clean milk. Use of oxytocin or any other hormone and drug should not be used to let down the milk. Milk should be stored at 4-6°C to prevent growth of bacteria and to maintain good quality. It should be transported to the factory or market as soon as possible to maintain its quality.

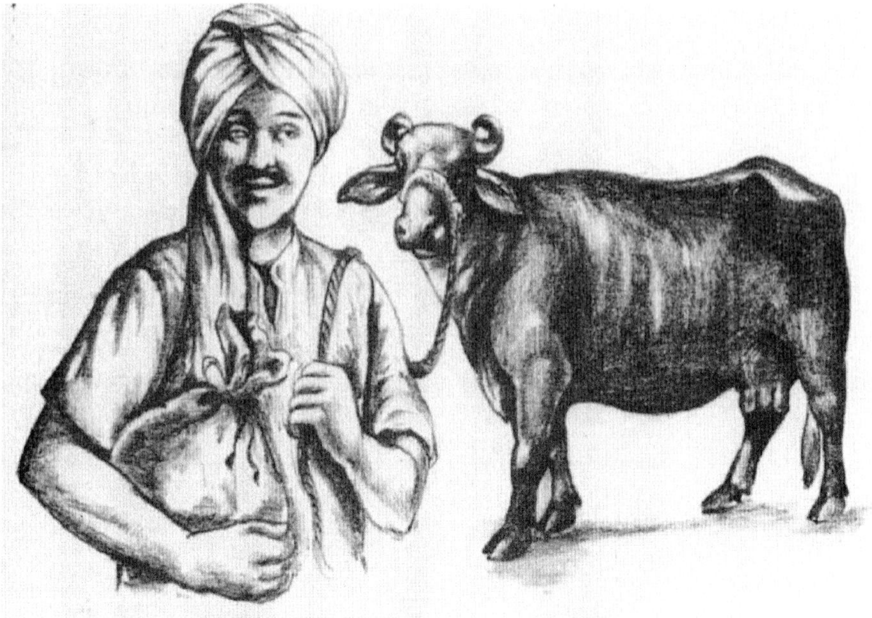

Getting involved in quality milk production is easy. All you have to do is make a commitment to get involved. An attitude for quality is an attitude for profit.

Examples for teaching clean milk production

Practical activities: Self learning activities

1. What does a swollen mammary gland indicate?
2. What should be the maximum time for milking the animal?
3. What type of environment is required for milking of animals?
4. What are the various changes in milk that indicate mastitis?
5. What are the factors that increase/stimulate let-down of milk in dairy animals?.
6. What is oxytocin?
7. What precautions need to be taken to prevent decline in milk yield during summer?
8. How can we prevent incidence of mastitis in a cow?

Practical activities

i) To understand the milk let-down mechanism, take a lactating cow. Do udder and teat message for 2-5 minutes. Observes the changes in teat and udder size before and after message.

ii) Find out the change in animal behavior during teat message and milking without and with concentrate mixture feeding.

iii) Keep the animals under tree, in houses with fan in summer, and observe the effect on milk yield.

Self assessment- questions with answers

Q1. Why keeping of milk production and health record is important?

Ans. The records are important to know about the daily milk yield changes, incidence of mastitis and total milk production by the animal in a month or complete lactation period.

Q2. What is the importance of oxyticn in let-down of milk in dairy animals?

Ans. Oxtycin hormone releases due to milking/ hand stimulus and causes let-down of milk in the udder.

Q3. What are the advantages of the machine milking?

Ans. Machine milking of animals results in clean milk production as milk flows directly from the teat to the milk collection tank (or in bucket). Thus there is no contamination of milk due to falling hairs, flies, dung, dirt and any other foreign particles.

Q4. What should be done to prevent contamination of milk during hand milking?

Ans. Milk should be filtered through a muslin cloth or sieve. The animal's udder, teat, milking place and milking bucket should also be clean.

Q5. What is the accurate method of hand milking?

Ans. Hand milking should be done by fisting method in which all hand fingers and palm is used. This method provides stimulus similar to calf suckling.

Q6. What type of milking bucket/pails is used in hand milking?

Ans. Milking pails should be made up of stainless steel or aluminum or galvanized iron.

Q7. Why proper method of milking should be adopted to milk the cows?

Ans. Wrong method of hand milking may result in teat injury, mastitis and low milk yield.

Q8. What type of precautions should be taken to clean the milking pails?

Ans. The crevices of pails should be cleaned with chemical like sodium hypo-chloride or teepol. Invert the pail after washing for complete drying. Milking pails should be of cylindrical shape to minimize entry of foreign particles in milk

Q9. What do you understand by the term CMT?

Ans. California mastitis test (CMT) is done to test the abnormal milk due to mastitis. Take 5 ml milk and add equal amount of CMT solution. Mix and observe the solution after 2-3 minutes for the following change.

A. No Change in consistency – Milk is normal

B. Little gel formation – Udder inflammation

C. Consistent gel formation – Mastitis milk

Q10. In what way the health of milker is related to clean milk production.

Ans. Milker should be healthy and should not have disease like cough, fever, TB and any other infectious disease.

Q11. What is the name of milk sugar?

Ans. Lactose is the only significant sugar found in milk.

Assignments Based on Unit

- What are the advantages of machine milking in animals?
- What do you understand by let-down of milk?
- Why cooling of milk is essential after milking?
- What are the important steps in clean milk production?
- What type of milking environment animals require for complete milking?
- What are factors that inhibit milk letdown in a cow?

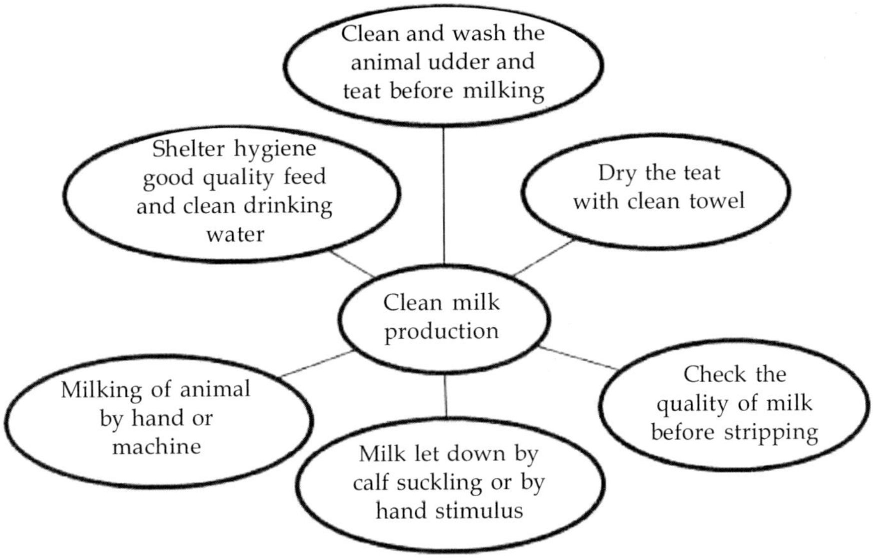

Requirements of clean milk production

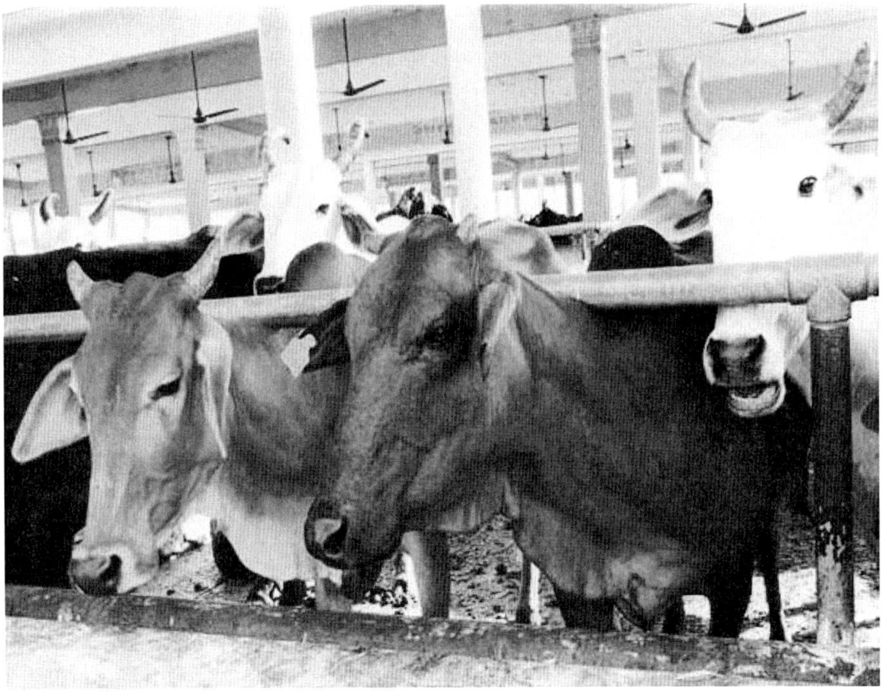

Photo. Use of fans to ameliorate heat stress in cows

❑❑❑

Chapter-28

Physiogenomic Aspects of Persistency of Lactation

The decline in milk yield after peak lactation in dairy animals are causes of considerable loss of income for the dairy farmer. Recent advances in understanding the control of the mammary cell population has revealed that a change in mammary cell number occurs due to imbalance between cell proliferation and cell removal. This is the principal cause of decline in milk production. Further persistency of lactation (the rate of decline in milk yield) with stage of lactation is strongly influenced by the rate of cell death by apoptosis in the lactating gland. Mammary apoptosis was first demonstrated during tissue involution after lactation, but has now been detected during lactation, in mammary tissue of lactating mice, goats and cattle. Factors that determine the rate of cell death by apoptosis are as yet poorly characterized, but include the frequency of milking in lactating goats. Nutrition and oxidative stress imposed by feed and the tissue's ability to deal with it also influence cell survival after peak lactation. However, molecular mechanisms controlling mammary cell survival (or otherwise) are yet poorly defined. There is considerable incentive to elucidate the determinants of mammary apoptosis and the factors controlling the dynamic balance between cell proliferation and cell death in the lactating mammary gland.

Milk production or lactation phenomenon starts at parturition and continues until the animal gets dry-off. Its evolution over time is characterised by a peculiar milk yield pattern generally known as lactation curve. The curve is characterised by an initial increasing phase from parturition till a maximum yield, followed by a declining phase after peak lactation generally 4-6 weeks in cattle with lowest at the end stage also known as dry off period. The whole lactation curve shape is broadly divided into two main components; i) which is generally characterized as regular and continuous with general or predictable pattern and ii) as random with unpredictable pattern in different animals. The first component is a direct consequence of the physiological processes which involves either synthesis and secretion of milk constituents in the mammary gland or direct transfer of certain constituents to mammary tissue from the blood stream. The second component is represented by several factors such as genetic make-up, feeding management, farming system, climate and health of the animal. In certain rare situations like rearing of animals on pasture-based feeding system, double lactation peaks have been observed in sheep and cattle which is of economic benefits to farmers. Animals with sharp decline or less persistency produce less milk and bears higher cost of milk production due to less efficiency of production. Increasing the milk production efficiency is often associated with impaired health and fertility in dairy cows. This led to the incorporation of functional traits into breeding to counteract this negative association.

Lactation persistency

Lactation persistency is defined as the ability of a cow to maintain a relatively constant milk yield throughout lactation, or the potential to continue producing milk at a high level after peak lactation. Better persistency is an indicative of low rate of decline in milk yield and lower decline in epithelial cells of mammary gland. Thus high lactation persistency is associated with a slow rate of decline in milk production, whereas low lactation persistency is associated with a rapid rate of decline. Cows with greater lactation persistency are more profitable than average cows when yield and lactation persistency are correlated. More persistent animal often utilize better feed and fodders, suffers less to stress and have more resistant to diseases with less reproduction failures.

Why to model lactation curve

On a dairy farm the pattern of milk yield across the year depicts the trend of a farm income and strong correlation with nutritive requirements of dairy animals. Attempts have been made to develop mathematical tools to accurately predict the milk yield in normal or mastitis animals during the year. It also helps to forecast future yield in a dairy farm. Another important field of application of lactation curve modelling is the genetic improvement of milk production traits. Lactation curve modelling address to the reconstruction of the regular and continuous component of the lactation pattern which is useful for management decision and research studies. The genetic merit of the animals via, random regression test day models can also be done. Estimation of lactation persistency can be grouped as *i.e.* mathematical models describing the lactation curve, based on ratios between total, partial, maximum or other yields, variation of yields in the course of the lactation and by application of random regression test day models.

Criteria based on mathematical models

Various mathematical models to fit lactation curves have been reviewed. The common aim of mathematical functions is to predict the test day yields, part lactation yields and environmental effects on the shape of lactation curves. The most simple model for a lactation curve is a linear regression of test day yields on days in milk but is not in conformity with lactation curve function since lactation curves for yield traits consist, dearly distinguishable for milk, ascending phase between calving and peak yield, constant production around peak yield and a descending part after peak yield. The regression coefficient could be viewed as a criterion of persistency. The Wood model is the most widely used function for the description of lactation curves because it considers the basic features of lactation curves with only three parameters such as average production, maximum production and day to maximum production.

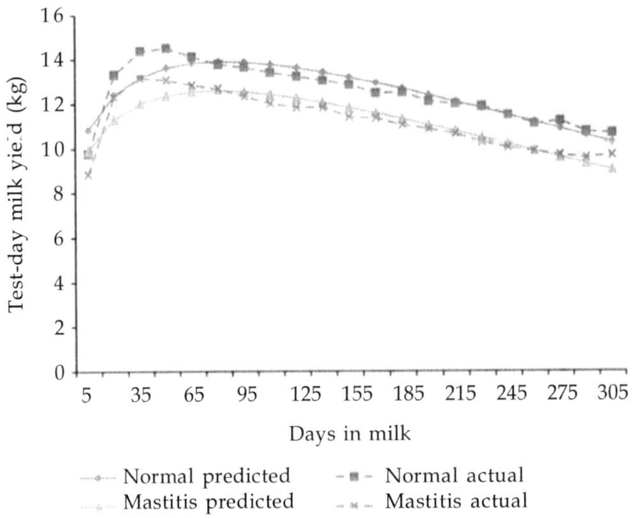

Figure. Comparison of the actual and predicted FTDMY of normal and mastitic Karan Fries cows in the first lactation.

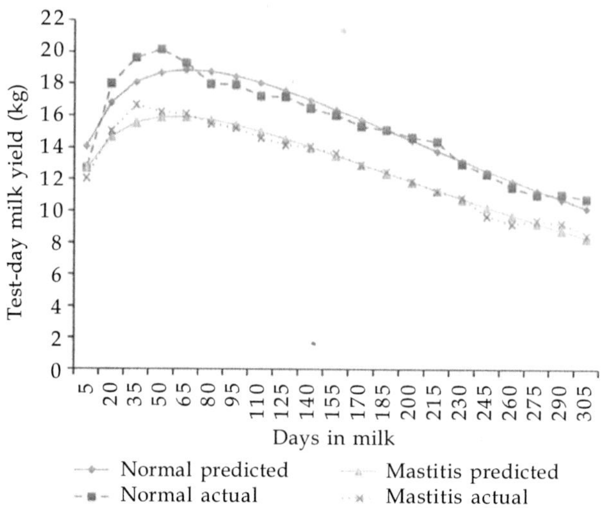

Figure. Comparison of the actual and predicted FTDMY of normal and mastitic Karan Fries cows in the fifth and above lactation.

Criteria based on ratio of yields

Persistency is the ratio between mean and peak yield or ratio of total yield during lactation to peak yield or ratio of 305-day lactation yield divided by peak yield multiplied by 305 days. In this criterion, higher values of milk yield are associated with higher persistency. Some authors used the ratio of peak yield divided by the average yield during lactation or in parts of the lactation. In these studies, higher values criterion are indicators of lower persistency. Another variant is the ratios of partial yields, namely the ratio of production in the second 100 days to that of the first 100 days and analogously the ratio of the last to the first trimester of lactation. These measurements became very popular due to their ease of computation and to compare ascending and descending phases of the lactation.

Criteria associated with the variation of test day yields

The standard deviation of test day yields during the lactation is used to measure persistency. The model considers variations of test day yields due to undesirable oscillations of the lactation curve. The distribution of this criterion is closer to a normal one than for other measurements of persistency. The limitation is that standard deviation of lactation yields is not independent of the total or average yield per day in the lactation. So, a modified criterion called yield variation measuring the variation of accumulated part-lactation yields and combining these values into an index was developed. Also square-root transformation of yield variation provides a persistency parameter that has a near perfect normal distribution.

Criteria derived from random regression test day models

The models take into account repeated measurements (test day and yields) within a lactation and are modelled partly by fixed regression coefficients, often nested in appropriate subgroups of the data (*e.g.* calving age and season) and partly by random regression coefficients associated with the animal's genetic effect and environmental effect, thus allowing for a covariance structure among the coefficients. Random regression models are used for analysis of repeated measurements. Random regression models estimate the shape of the genetic lactation curve or genetic persistency for every animal by fitting the curve using daily breeding values individually for each lactation, with simultaneous correction. The model has advantages of accuracy of genetic evaluations, genetic persistency and better understanding of the genetics of lactation.

Factors affecting persistency

Non-genetic factors

Parity: Generally it has been found that first lactation animals are more persistent than later lactations. First parturition animals possess continuous body and udder development. Due to this reason primiparous have low milk production capacity and have higher persistency as compared to pluriparous cows. This could also be attributed to more number of secretory cells in mammary gland, which maintain their secretory activity for a longer duration in first lactation compared to subsequent lactations where amount of milk secretion by each secretory cell is increased however, it fails to maintain their secretory activity for a longer duration and finally get sloughed off at early stage of lactation.

Age at Calving: Age at calving have least effect within parity. The reducing trend in persistency with increase in age at first calving is attributed to negative relationship between persistency and yield. It is well known that yield increases with age at calving. From this a more developed mammary gland of an old animal should also lead to sharper peak of the lactation curve.

Season of calving

Different regions of the world have their specific environmental conditions, feeding and mangemental practices. A strong seasonal effect is observed in a pasture based feeding system whereas regions having less climatic variations, the effect of season is negligible on persistency of lactation. The higher persistency in rainy and autumn calvers is due to regular availability of green fodder and conducive weather conditions. In tropical countries like India animals have lesser persistency during summer due to more heat stress and green fodder scarcity. Thus availability of green fodders and the nutrients at different stages of lactation influences the persistency of lactation.

Gestation: The status of pregnancy (> 5 months) significantly influences persistency of lactation. Pregnancy status can be accounted for by including in the model number of days open, days in calf or calving interval. The cows which conceive early are subjected to a higher metabolic stress since it coincides with the peak yield. Such cows exhibit depressing effect on persistency of lactation. Thus cows with a superior reproductive performance exhibit low persistency. First lactation cows with high persistency tend to have better conception within 56 days after their first insemination (genetic correlation of 32%). There is a higher persistency in days open between 60 to 150 than early or late conceivers in Sahiwal cows. The effect of service period on persistency may reflect the replenishment of body tissues after parturition. The changes in endocrine profile in early pregnancy mainly progesterone leading to lowering of persistency.

Days to attain peak yield

Maximum average of persistency was obtained for Sahiwal cows having days to attain peak yield between 110-120 days and the persistency was minimum for cows having 33-43 days to attain peak yield. Cows taking lesser days to attain peak-yield were lesser persistent than the cows taking longer days to attain peak-yield. It also reveal that cows taking higher number of days to attain peak yield face lesser metabolic stress in early lactation than the cows attaining peak yield earlier.

Genetic parameters for persistency

Heritability and repeatability of lactation persistency

The heritability estimate of persistency of milk yield has been moderate to high ranging from 0.03 to 0.59. The high variability indicated that this trait is significantly influenced by genetic factors and can be improved through selection. Repeatability of persistency in consecutive lactation is very low. Genetic correlation between persistencies for identical traits in successive lactations is around 0.30. A strong genetic relationship between milk and protein yield has been found than that between milk and fat yield. Reports are available for a correlation of 0.80 and 0.90 between milk and fat persistency and milk and protein persistency.

Genetic and phenotypic correlation with 305 days milk yield

An important characteristic of the persistency measure is its correlation with the 305-days milk yield. The high persistent lactation cows leads to longer production periods. Genetic correlations range 0.2-0.6 between persistency of milk yield and FL305DMY. Cows with a high genetic level for persistency often have lower genetic level for milk production.

Persistency and first lactation peak-yield

Genetically lactation persistency is positively and negatively correlated with peak yield ranging from -0.6-0.9. The phenotypic correlations between persistency of milk yield and FLPY range between -0.2 to 0.8.

Persistency and calving interval

Genetically an antagonistic relationship exists between persistency and reproductive performance. Poor reproductive performance leads to economic losses due to reduced milk production and prolong calving interval. Studies analysing the genetics of lactation persistency should always account for influence of gestation. Secondly, bio-economic models for optimal management strategies have to consider the two-fold relationship between persistency and reproductive performance. Cows of higher persistency have a flatter lactation curve which is an indicator of lower metabolic stress and superior reproductive performance.

Persistency and longevity

The length of productive life is probably the most important trait in cattle breeding. The longer animals remain productive in a herd, the fewer animals are required. The relationship between persistency and longevity needs to be analysed. Until now, little has been known in this field. The correlation between the breeding value of persistency and the relative breeding value of longevity is 0.06. The high scores for lactation persistency are actually associated with a shorter herd life.

Persistency and health disorders

Cows that start their first lactation with a difficult calving will tend to have a more persistent lactation (genetic correlation of 43%) due to poorer start of lactation and peak yield compared to easy calvers. There is an unfavourable genetic correlation among persistency and metabolic diseases. Primiparous and multiparous cows, which develop postpartum metabolic disorders (ketosis, milk fever, displaced abomasum) and periparturiant reproductive disorders (metritis, retained placenta, and ovarian cysts) attain peak yield at later days and have flatter lactation curves for milk fat, and protein yields. Disease incidence significantly influences lactation persistency rather than persistency affecting disease occurrence. Mastitis in early lactation tends to produce highly persistent lactations more often in multiparous cows than primiparous cows. However, mastitis tends to reduce milk yield persistency due to less milk, fat, and protein yield persistencies. The effect of lameness on milk, fat, and protein yield persistencies is negligible. To increase persistency, indicators of female fertility have to be included in the genetic evaluation to reduce undesirable side effects on fertility in cows

Relationship of persistency with body condition and milk SCC

The relationship between lactation persistency and recovery of body reserves in late lactation are favourable. Persistency is positively correlated (r=0.28) with BCS. Cows with high lactation persistency tend to be healthy and recover body reserves well in late lactation. The relationships till date are phenotypically based, and persistency based on genetic relationships needs to be explored. A negative correlation of 0.123 between lactation persistency and SCC reveal that persistency of lactation improves with a moderate decrease in

SCC. Thus cows with a high cell count have a reduced persistency of milk yield.

Genes related to persistency

The endocrine regulation and physiology of milk production has been elucidated extensively but the genetics that underlie these dynamics are still uncovered. Few studies have estimated exact gene and marker effects at different time-points during lactation. In most livestock studies, the change in additive genetic variation over time was analyzed mainly for body weight and milk yield in dairy cattle, sheep, and goats. However, most of the studies used either no marker information or only a few markers on selected chromosomes to conduct their analyses. The described effects of the DGAT1 gene, with antagonistic impacts on milk yield and fat content, were shown to be detectable only after 40 days of lactation. This late effect points to a possible utilization of DGAT1 in changing the persistency of milk production. Markers around the casein genes had strongest effects in early lactation, which is confirmed by the higher protein content in colostrum milk. In general, the highest variation in associated loci occurs in early and late lactation.

Future research

Persistency is affected by management strategies that are often not recorded in the data. Management strategies for feeding in the course of the lactation and policies for the handling of the reproductive performance are likely to mask the real persistency that may be desirable as a trait for selection. Future studies on the genetics of persistency should explore the interaction of geneticists and physiologists confounded with the problem of metabolic stress. Research needs to be carried out on how much milk a cow can produce without inducing an energy deficiency under natural feeding conditions and how much milk a cow should produce to be still profitable for the farmer by using appropriate genetics model curve?

(Contributed by: Mohsin Ayoub, Mohammad Rayees, Aasif Ahmad, Showkat Ahmad)

❑❑❑

Chapter-29

Markers to Augment Animal Productivity

India is one of the world's five largest producers of livestock and poultry meat. The livestock sector from the economic point of view contributes 28% and 5% of the country's agricultural and total gross domestic product, respectively. The world's largest bovine populations of 199 million cattle, which constitute about 14.7% of the world's total cattle population exist in India. India has become largest producer of milk (144.5 billion kg) in 2014-2015 due to advancement in R & D activities and use of elite germ plasm. Buffalo and cattle contribute about 55% and 45% of the total milk production in our country. Inspite of high milk production, the average productivity of Indian cow is very low (2.5kg/d) than that of developed countries.

The overall sexual reproduction processes are well documented in cows and buffaloes, however molecular and genetic basis of reproduction is less defined. The complexity and transient nature of specific reproductive processes are the basic limitation concerning their molecular basis. Considerable, improvements have been made in determining the economic traits like growth or feed efficiency using genetic and selection management advances, however measures to improve reproductive efficiency still needs more attention in most of the livestock species. There is a need of identification and characterization of specific genes and genomic regions which have a direct role in regulation of reproductive processes. Understanding the genetic control of female reproductive performance would offer the opportunity to utilize natural variation and improve selective breeding programme. In the last decades, two main approaches have been widely applied for this goal in different domestic species: Candidate gene studies and Genome scans. Both approaches have been useful respectively in the identification of associations of specific gene polymorphisms or genomic regions with reproductive traits. More recently the study of genome at structural (SNP chips) and functional (expression microarrays) levels offer new possibilities to study genetic variation and metabolic pathways influencing reproductive efficiency. SNPs are the fundamental unit of genetic variation and are used as markers because of their abundance and association with economic traits in cattle. Variations in DNA in a single nucleotide may help to predict response to certain drugs, susceptibility to environment and risk of developing diseases. The inheritance of disease genes within families can also be tracked. Identification of markers of milk quality and production traits, disease resistance and thermo-tolerance will ensure better health and productivity. Also, markers for fertility and carcass quality traits could be used for preferred growth in cattle.

What is molecular marker?

A molecular marker is a DNA fragment in the genome and can be defined as a genetic marker. This marker is used in identifying partial DNA sequence in an unknown DNA pool. Several types of DNA molecular markers have been explored since 1980 to evaluate genetic diversity. In 1990, Scientists in the USA initiated use of rapid amplification of polymorphic DNA (RAPD) markers and amplified fragment length polymorphisms. Following this markers like restriction fragment length polymorphism (RFLP) mini-satellites polymerase chain reaction (PCR) based markers [microsatellites and single nucleotide polymorphisms (SNPs)] have been used. However, major challenge is how to identify gene markers that control phenotypic variation in the target traits. Genetic markers have been classified based on visually evaluated traits (morphological and productive traits), gene product (biochemical markers) and DNA analysis (molecular markers). Molecular marker refers to specific DNA variation between individuals like insertions, deletions, translocations, duplications and point mutations. These can be measured in blood or tissue sample and are not confounded by environment, pleiotropic, or epistatic effects.

Molecular marker study

Reproductive technologies such as artificial insemination, multiple ovulation, and embryo transfer led to considerable improvement in animal productivity. Traditional breeding techniques in dairy cattle take many years and do not efficiently take into account all sources of genetic variability. Due to low heritable or late-expressed traits. In this regard molecular marker application address the problems associated with selection of genetically superior animals and to improve disease resistance.

Advantages and limitations of molecular markers

Genetic marker have wide range of immediate applications like parentage determination, estimation of genetic distance, twin zygosity and freemartinism, sexing of preimplantation embryos and disease carrier identification, gene mapping and marker-assisted selection. Molecular markers can easily be used as reference points in transgenic breeding and in identification of animals with specific transgenes. Thus improvement in livestock health and productivity could be achieved by use of molecular markers in the near future.

Molecular marker used in cattle genetic research

Two major categories of molecular markers have been identified i) hybridization-based and ii) PCR-based markers. Various families of hypervariable repetitive DNA sequences like mini-satellites and microsatellites can be subjected to hybridization to reveal DNA fingerprinting. The PCR-based markers are arbitrary PCR assays. Cleaved amplified polymorphic sequence, allele specific PCR, PCR amplification of specific alleles, sequence length polymorphism and targeted microsatellite site have been classified in sequence-targeted PCR assays category. Arbitrary PCR assays include RAPD, RAPD-RFLP, and microsatellite-primed PCR. Microsatellites are the potential markers that could be used for livestock genetic studies due to their easy application using PCR and electrophoresis. Hypervariable microsatellite in the bovine steroid 21-hydroxylase gene is a classic example wherein dinucleotide blocks may be an abundant source of DNA polymorphism in cattle. SNPs gained high popularity due to biallelic type of marker and are most abundant of all marker systems in animal and plant genomes. Besides this SNPs have genetically high stability and amenability in automated analysis.

Markers of quality milk production

Phenotypic and biochemical markers have been frequently used to identify an animal with high genetic merit for economic traits in cattle. In the recent years, the research priority has been focused on identification of molecular markers of economic importance that are widely accepted. Around 344 quantitative trait loci (QTL) associated with milk traits and 71 with mastitis related traits has been identified. Association between DNA polymorphism and milk production traits have been studied for prolactin; leptin; diacylglycerol acyltransferase (DGAT1); stearoyl-CoA desaturase; bovine leukocytic antigen (BoLA)-DRB3 gene, growth hormone receptor gene, casein α s1 (CSN1S1) gene; ATP-binding cassette, subfamily G, member 2 (ABCG2) gene; protease inhibitor gene; osteopontin gene; proliferator-activated receptor gamma, coactivator (CoA) 1 α gene; growth hormone (GH) gene; signal transducer and activator of transcription (STAT) 1 oxidized low density lipoprotein receptor 1; cytochrome P450, subfamily XI B, polypeptide 1; fatty acid synthase; caspase recruitment domain-containing protein 15; bovine K-casein gene CSN3, thyroglobulin gene; â-lactoglobulin gene; POU class 1 homeobox 1; STAT5A; and stearoyl CoA desaturase. Fourteen major milk proteins showing variability at DNA level have been reported in cattle. Milk proteins such as β-casein and Fourteen major milk proteins showing variability at DNA level κ-casein have proven valuable in assessing the milk quality and lactation of dairy cattle.

Table. Markers of lactogenic parameters in dairy cattle

S.No.	Polymorphic genes	Linked traits
1.	PRL (prolactin)	Milk production performance overall
2.	LEP (leptin)	Better milk yield with good energybalance and fertility
3.	DGAT1 (diacylglycerol O-acyltransferase 1)	Milk yield and composition
4.	SCD1 (stearoyl-CoA desaturase)	Milk fatty acid composition
5.	BoLA-DRB3 (Bos taurus major histocompatibility complex, class II, DRB3)	Somatic cell count and altered milkproduction traits
6.	GHR (growth hormone receptor)	Milk yield and composition
7.	CSN1S1 (casein α s1)	Milk protein expression
8.	ABCG2 (ATP-binding cassette, subfamily G, member 2)	Milk yield and composition
9.	PI (protease inhibitor)	Milk production and reproduction traits
10.	Osteopontin/SPP1 (secreted phosphoprotein 1)	Milk production traits

11.	PPARGC1A (proliferator-activated receptor gamma, coactivator 1α)	Milk fat synthesis
12.	GH (growth hormone)	Milk production traits
13.	STAT1 (signal transducer and activatorof transcription 1)	Milk protein synthesis and fat metabolism
14.	OLR1 (oxidized low density lipoproteinreceptor 1)	Milk fat yield and fat percentage
15.	CYP11B1 (cytochrome P450, subfamily XI B, polypeptide 1)	Milk production traits
16.	FASN (fatty acid synthase)	Milk fat
17.	CARD15/NOD2 (nucleotide-binding oligomerization domain containing 2)	Milk production traits
18.	CSN3 (casein k)	Milk production related traits
19.	TG (thyroglobulin)	Intramuscular fat and milk production traits
20.	LGB (β-lactoglobulin)	Milk protein concentration
21.	PIT 1/POU1F1 (POU class 1 homeobox 1)	Milk yield and productive life
22.	STAT5A (signal transducer and activator of transcription 5A)	Milk composition
23.	SCD (stearoyl CoA desaturase)	Milk production traits

The molecular markers for prolactin, leptin, DGAT1 and ABCG2 genes have association with milk traits, while leptin is considered as a powerful biomolecule for enhancing productivity in animals. This hormone have pivotal role in lactogenesis, colostrum secretion, galactopoiesis, and immunity to mastitis. Due to this reason it is an important candidate gene for genetic studies. C/BspEI/T and C/HphI/T polymorphisms of leptin gene are associated with milk protein percentage and C/HphI/T locus of leptin is associated with Solid non fat percentage. Prolactin hormone is another potential quantitative trait locus affecting milk production traits in dairy cattle. Based on the SNP analysis, CHBP2 and diplotype H2H8 of prolactin could be useful genetic markers in a selection of milk production traits in Holstein dairy cattle. DGAT1 polymorphism is now recognized as an important candidate marker for fat content and ABCG2 gene has significant effect on milk fat and protein. Microsatellite markers have been found to be fruitful in determining the specific molecular markers on milk quality e.g., QTL such as BTA6 have an effect on milk fat and protein. The available QTL database of cattle could now be used to integrate information from different sources to find out the causative sites for the QTL for all probable variation to elucidate the economic traits

Molecular markers of fertility

More emphasis is now given in mapping and identifying genes that regulate reproductive traits due to sex-limitedness and low heritability of reproductive traits. The role of genes that relate to bovine follicle stimulating hormone receptor; luteinizing hormone/ choriogonadotropin receptor; bovine inhibin á; bovine progesterone receptor; and growth differentiation factor 9 needs to explored. These genes can be used as potential markers for super ovulation response due to association with the total number of ova produced and number of transferable embryos. Similarly polymorphism C/NruI/T of bovine leptin gene has association with age at first service and age at first calving. It has been reported that fertilization failure or embryogenesis failures are potentially of seminal origin. Molecular markers in candidate genes like cation channel of sperm 1, sperm-specific NHE, A kinase, anchor protein 4, pyruvate kinase, cytochrome oxidase, reproductive homeobox 5, cysteine rich secretory protein 2, phosphatidylethanolamine binding protein 1, Doppel, tissue inhibitor of metalloproteinase have been found for assessing semen quality and bull fertility. Protamine 1 and 2 genes express differentially among normal and motility impaired semen of Frieswal bulls.

Table. Reproductive performance parameters and their markers in dairy animals

S.No.	Molecular Markers	Reproductive traits
01.	BTA7 and BTA10	Calving and fertility traits
02.	FSHB	Quality of fresh and frozen semen
03.	Cocaine and amphetamine-regulatedtranscript (CART)	Follicle health status
04.	IGF-I	Follicular development and ovulation
05.	FSHB, Per1	Folliculogenesis and oogenesis
06.	Survivin	Embryo quality
07.	Production of prolactin-related protein 1 (PRP-1)	Implantation
08.	bPRP-1	Trophoblastic cell differentiation and pregnancy diagnosis
09.	Bovine chromosome 3 (BTA3), QTL-F-Fert - BTA3	Repeat breading and female fertility

10.	IGF-IR	Productive and reproductive traits
11.	STAT5A	Fertilization and early embryonic development, initiation of pregnancy, milk production and health traits
12.	FSHR	Regulation of ovarian function
13.	Uterine serpins (SERPINA14)	Pregnancy
14.	CYP19	Anestrum
15.	FSHR, IGF-IR and STAT5A	Calving interval
16.	Amphiregulin (AREG)	Embryonic attachment
17.	STAR	Regulation of steroidogenesis
18.	INHBA and INHBB, FST and ACNA	Different stages of seminiferous epithelial cycle regulated spermatogenesis
19.	Follistatin (FST)	Modulate a range of testicular actions of activin
20.	Inhibin beta B	Sperm concentration trait
21.	Osteopontin (OPN)	Bull fertility, sperm-binding and fertilization
22.	Cytochrome P450 aromatase (arom P450)	Sperm quality and motility
23.	IGF-IR	Productive and reproductive traits

The research studies during the last one decade have clearly identified number of molecular markers to improve the milk production performance and their association with disease, productive and reproductive traits in cattle and buffaloes. The essence of using genetic markers in breeding programs is that they mark chromosomal regions (and sometimes individual genes) and make it possible to follow the inheritance of these regions from parents to offspring. Thus measure of polymorphisms at loci along with microsatellite markers and microarray technology has great potential to augment cattle health and productivity as a whole in the years to come.

(Contributed by: Mohammad Rayees)

❑❑❑

Chapter-30

Milk with A1 and A2 β-casein Protein

Milk from dairy cow is considered as nature's perfect food. It is an important source of nutrients including high quality proteins, carbohydrates and micronutrients. Milk contains about 95% proteins like caseins and whey proteins. Among caseins, the beta casein has excellent nutritional balance of amino acids and is the second most abundant protein in milk. Several experiments have demonstrated different variants of β-casein in milk evolved over many years due to mutation and selective breeding for higher milk production. There are 15 known variants of β -casein including A1 and A2. Beta casein-A1 differs from A2 by one amino acid at 67th position. There is a substitution of histidine (A1) in place of proline in A2 milk. It has been postulated that A1 β-casein is more susceptible to hydrolysis by digestive enzymes to produce beta-casomorphin7 (BCM7) which is an active deca-peptide. A school of thought claims this peptide to be a causative agent of many human health problems while others talk about its beneficial effects. However, both types of milk are considered to be safer for adults and children. BCM must be released in intestine after consuming A1 milk, for studying its biological effects on heart or brain, but there are no reports to show that BCM is released in the intestine after consuming A1 milk. There is no evidence that BCM is absorbed intact in the intestine from where it enters into the blood circulation. It is noteworthy that the intestine of a healthy human can absorb tri-peptides at the most. As per physiology of digestion the long chain of BCM should be broken in the intestine into smaller peptides before absorption. Larger peptides can cross intact only in the intestine of new-born infants with severe intestinal diseases. There are published reports that BCM and other beta caseins have beneficial effects in humans. BCM contributes to the production of mucin in intestine which has protective function and prevents kidney complications in diabetic patients.

Protein chain showing amino acids in A1 and A2 beta-casein

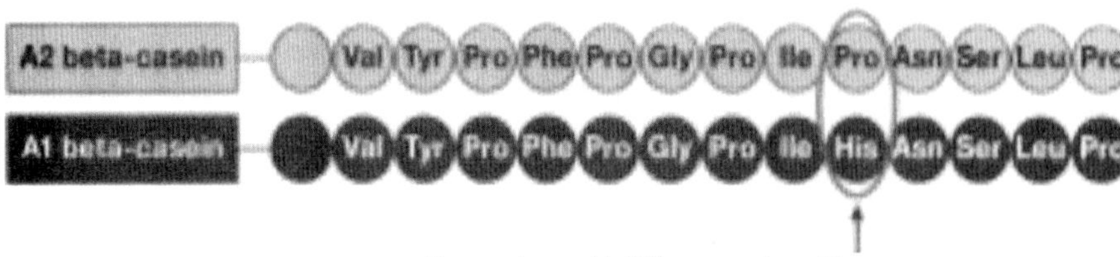
A2 beta-casein
Val Tyr Pro Phe Pro Gly Pro Ile Pro Asn Ser Leu Pro
A1 beta-casein
Val Tyr Pro Phe Pro Gly Pro Ile His Asn Ser Leu Pro

One amino acid difference at position 67 in the protein chain

Research studies need to confirm about the adverse effects of BCM7 in Infants having immature GI tract, whereas adults gather the biological activity locally on the intestinal brush boarder. Initial studies on Indigenous cow (Tharparkar, Sahiwal, Red Sindhi of Zebu type), buffaloes and exotic cows (taurine type) have revealed that A1 allele is frequently present in exotic cattle while Indian native cows and buffaloes have only A2 allele. Artificial insemination of cows with the semen of such bulls multiplied A1 gene frequency over the years. It has been shown that A1/A2 frequency is not breed-specific but area-specific. A1 frequency in Holstein Friesen breed is said to be very high (>90%) in North America and North Europe but A2 frequency of the same breed is very high (97 %) in Germany. However, A1 frequencies of this breed ranges between (40–65%) in other countries. According to National Bureau of Animal Genetic Resources (NBAGR), A2 gene frequency in Indian breeds of cattle is around 98%, whereas all the buffalo breeds are A2A2 type. Screening of samples from HF, Jersey and crossbred bulls in India have confirmed that these were predominantly carrying A2 allele. It has been clarified that even in crossbred cow population, the most predominant gene is A2.

Controversy over A1and A2

The harmful effects of A1 milk have been reported in media around the world without any concrete scientific research evidence. It is known fact that A1 milk might increase the risk of certain diseases but cannot cause a disease on its own. The research survey conducted in Australia during 1990 found strong association between high A1 β-casein consumption and coronary heart disease (CHD) and type-I diabetes mellitus. This association was stronger in high altitude countries like North America and Europe. India is not a high altitude country and it has different socio-economic attributes too. So these results cannot be applied to India. European Food Safety Authority has already rebutted the claims about the harmful effects of A1 type casein in milk. Countries like Sweden, Austria, Iceland, Canada and Germany have much higher A1 beta casein consumption than France and Australia but the mortality rates due to CHD were only 70-80 per Lakh people. Although A1 beta casein consumption have not changed in USA, Australia, Switzerland during the last decade but CHD mortality has dropped too much. Similarly Type-I diabetes mellitus is caused by the complex interactions between many factors in the developed countries.

Conclusion

There is hardly a publication to prove an association between CHD and BCM interactions in humans; but a study in rabbit reported binding of BCM with specific opioid receptors and neural cells leading to autism, schizophrenia and other neurological disorders. However there is no credible evidence till date to suggest that consumption of A1 milk is related to CHD, type-I diabetes mellitus and autism. Moreover, no scientific evidence suggests that A2 type milk could provide protection from these diseases. In view of the scanty literature and research studies and growing public concern about A1 and A2 milk there is a need to conduct more research studies before coming up with reasonable recommendations on A2 milk.

A1 and A2 milk can only be identified through genotyping using RFLP-PCR test. This test is complicated and not available everywhere. DNA is extracted from the test samples and A1/A2 probes are used to identify the genotype. The traders may cheat people as the test for judging A1/A2 is not only expensive but time consuming as well. Indian breeds of cows are much superior to exotic breeds due to their genetic characters such as heat tolerance, disease resistance and longevity. There is a need to conserve the best genetic characters and multiply only those animals which are superior in performance.

❑❑❑

Chapter-31

Genetic Engineering to Improve Milk Quality

The genetic improvement of livestock has been achieved traditionally through the application of principles of quantitative genetics and animal breeding. Milk production in dairy cattle has increased tremendously due to the genetic selection by artificial insemination. However, traditional animal breeding with new techniques of marker assisted selection could be more effective in the genetic improvement of our livestock. The arrival of modern biotechnological tools has opened new avenues for the improvement of milk production.

The biotechnology like artificial insemination and embryo transfer have been used successfully for last many years for genetic improvement of livestock. Currently it deals with more of molecular biology based techniques such as gene cloning and genetic engineering. Transgenic sheep, goats and cattle have been produced worldwide with these technologies. However, efficiency of producing transgenic ruminants is low and the costs are very high. In order to transfer a gene to the progeny of transgenic animal, it should be sexually mature and then complete a gestation which takes time. A nucleus from the recently fertilized ovum is the most common method to produce a genetically engineered livestock, although very few microinjected embryos produce transgenic animals. Biotechnology can be used to improve the genetic quality of livestock either by transferring new genetic material or disseminating the desirable traits via cloning of an animal. It has become possible to modify proteins now and have them secreted into the milk of a transgenic mammal. Such proteins have potential to improve the quality of milk and these are beneficial for the dairy industry.The genes encoding these proteins are transmitted through normal inheritance and the animals produce the proteins only in their milk during lactation. These new genes can be propagated in the dairy cattle population by use of embryo transfer, artificial insemination, in vitro fertilization and cloning.

Genetic Improvement through Cloning

Nuclear donors may be taken from transgenic fetal fibroblasts and engineered from connective tissue cells to clone calves and goat kids. The adult cells have also been used successfully for cloning the animals which can give rise to new dimensions in the genetic improvement of dairy animals. It is possible to produce a dairy cow capable of synthesizing milk with high protein content. This is an important feature for making cheese. Similarly it is also possible to produce a cow through cloning that has lower percentage of saturated fat, since it is beneficial for humans. Although selective breeding from an animal may not succeed always but selective breeding from a herd of cloned animals have more chances to succeed. Dairy industry may have potential impacts of genetic improvements on milk production. Cloning can be used to produce high yielding dairy cows. Artificial insemination has eliminated the need to clone elite bulls. While an elite cow is able to produce only a few offspring with the help of embryo transfer technology, the cloning has got an ability to increase the intensity of genetic selection. The current artificial insemination industry may be replaced by certain private companies in future for selling the clones of top dairy stock.

Improved livestock

The main aim of genetic engineering is to produce a livestock with altered traits such as disease resistance, better growth rate and milk composition. Gene constructs are the genes designed to express directly or indirectly various growth factors and change body composition. The majority of these transgenes expressed growth hormone; although other constructs based on GH release and insulin-like growth factor have also been used. Milk protein genes have been cloned from many animals. These transgenes are developmentally-correct, but their levels of expression can vary. Many private companies have produced transgenic cows, sheep, goats and pigs, targeting transgenic expression to the mammary gland with the aim of isolating high-value pharmaceutical proteins from milk.

It is possible to add a new gene or alter the existing genes to change the properties and composition of milk. A transgenic mice has been produced which expresses human lysozyme or a modified bovine casein in the milk. It has led to the change in the physical and functional properties of milk proteins, including decreased micelle size and increased gel strength. The production of human lysozyme in the milk of transgenic mice also increased the antimicrobial properties of the milk, which could reduce infections in the mammary gland of cows. It also help to eliminate unwanted pathogens in the human gut especially during consumption of milk. So the genetic engineering can be used to improve the livestock either by altering milk to improve its functionality in human health or by reducing the environmental pollution due to animal rearing. It is also possible to delete the genes responsible for certain diseases like mad cow disease.

Milk improvements: It is possible to bring about the variations in the composition and functionality associated with milk proteins, by over expression, deletion or addition of mutated form of major milk protein genes so that a desirable quality of cheese may be produced. The presence of 10% to 20% altered casein in milk produced by a transgenic cow can increase proteolysis and promote faster ripening of cheese. The genetically engineered dairy cows are able to produce healthier milk and more cheese yields as well as a wide variety of other milk products. The experiments are also being conducted to improve the nutritional and antimicrobial properties of milk. The research has demonstrated that human lysozyme is able to maintain antimicrobial activity when expressed as a transgene in mice. Trials are underway to add other naturally occurring human milk proteins with antimicrobial properties and genes to change the fatty-acid composition of milk so that it is good for the human heart. Such dairy cows with transgenes have great potential and could become available in the coming years! As a result of this, there will be separate herds for fluid milk production and those with the milk suited for cheese production. The antimicrobial properties of lysozyme-containing milk for drinking may interfere with the microbes used in cheese and yogurt production.

Environmental protection: Dairy and Livestock production units need to reduce the amount of minerals excreted by animals because the digestive processes of livestock can be inefficient and compounds like phosphates are being added to feed at levels exceeding the dietary requirements. These minerals accumulate at elevated levels in surface as well as groundwater which may damage the aquatic life and pollute the drinking water. The enzymes like phytase may be added to increase the efficiency of feed additives or the amount of phosphate in the feed can be reduced. Phytase enzymes decrease the amount of phosphate to be excreted and thus a better environment can be created. However application of cloning and genetic engineering technology to livestock raises a number of important issues.

Integration of a transgene into population: It is forecasted that transgenic animals could become useful in livestock production in coming 20 years. The transgene must be transferred to core breeding herds in the beginning and then the herds must undergo selection to optimize performance. It could be possible for transgenes to affect the traits like growth, body composition and reproduction. However introduction of a transgene into livestock will be very expensive due to the higher cost of breeding.

Genetic diversity and inbreeding: There is apotential concern that the use of cloned or genetically engineered animals may lead to reductions in the genetic diversity or increased inbreeding among livestock. However, such problems are not encountered when conventional breeding techniques are used. If cloned animals without any genetic variation are used properly within the context of a selective breeding program, then inbreeding could be easily minimized. The same is true for transgenic animals produced by microinjection, which are more inbred than the population at large. Maintenance of genetic diversity is necessary to allow future improvements through breeding for improved production and health.

Acceptance by the industry: The acceptance of genetic engineered animals by industry as well as the use of cloning to reproduce superior female, will depend upon the economic incentives. If the cost of stock or loss in selection progress is greater than the return to the producer through increased efficiencies or income over a reasonable period, producers will not use these technologies. In case the transgene results in new products, such as antimicrobial milk or moth-resistant wool, then producer would probably need to obtain a premium price to convert the production flock or herd to the new genotype. As with antimicrobial milk, the introduction of some new genotypes may lead to segmenting the industry and creating special uses for different populations of animals so that new "breeds" could be established. The acceptance of such genetically modified animals by industry and the farmers will depend upon the fact whether consumers are prepared to buy their milk and milk products.

Consumer acceptance

There is a lot of debate in European countries over the use of genetically modified crops. However, a number of genetically modified crops have been approved by the US for commercial use. There may be similar public debate on the introduction of genetically modified livestock. There are concerns on decreasing genetic diversity and the safety of genetically modified foods for human consumption. The issue is also related to the animal ethics and welfare. Since the growth-enhancing transgenes in animals may affect production traits rather than the quality of the final product, therefore consumers may not get any direct benefits. It is also possible that consumer may reject the same due to "no direct benefits" to them.

It is much easier to produce transgenic livestock through the cloning of genetically engineered animals yet the efficiency of its improvement is low and costs are high. Attention has to be given to avoid inbreeding during the production of transgenic animals. The mammary gland and the milk protein systems are robust and can be altered to use a variety of different proteins with normal functioning. These systems can be changed to produce desirable changes in the functional and antimicrobial properties of milk. While milk can be genetically modified easily, many important production traits like growth require genetic modification of basic metabolic systems. Researchers are optimistic about the future of transgenic animals. This technology will result in genetically modified more efficient and healthier than the current livestock. Although the low efficiency of current genetic engineering technology is a limiting factor, the need to carry out selection to optimize the performance of transgenic production animals may be an even greater limiting factor in the development of commercial herds. Public awareness needs to be created so that the consumers may fully understand the nature of these genetic modifications.

❑❑❑

APPENDIX-I

Objective Type Questions

Model Objective Type Questions I

Q1. Following two species of the primitive mammals represent many extinct species that were egg layers;

a) Duck bill platypus b) Spiny ant-eater or echidna

c) Both a and b d) None

Q2. One of the following **stage** does not relate to fetal mammary gland development stages;

a) Mammary streak b) Mammary band

c) Mammary bud d) Mammary involution

Q3. The basic unit of the alveolus is;

a) Mayo epithelial cell b) Epithelial cell

c) Histocytes d) None

Q4. During lactation mammary gland have,

a) 50% parenchyma and 50% Stroma
b) 70% parenchyma ad 30% Stroma
c) 80% parenchyma ad 20% Stroma
d) 90% parenchyma and 10%Stroma

Q5. Tissue culture of mammary gland have not been very successful due to ;

a) Quick death of epithelial cells
b) Poor growth of epithelial cells
c) Death of fibroblasts
d) Both a and b

Q6. Measurement of the following enables the researchers to determine connective tissue of mammary gland in toto;

a) DNA b) RNA

c) HYdroxyproline d) All the above

Q7. The mammary epithelial cells acquires capability to synthesize milk when one of following hormone concentration is less;

a) Estrogen b) Prolactin

c) Progesterone d) GH

Q8. The cells of the ectoderm get thickened on the ventral surface of embryo and forms mammary band at;

a) 30 days of age b) 40days of age

c) 50 days of age d) 60 days ofage

Q9. Mammary bud is formed when embryo is about;

a) 1.1cm long b) 2.1 cm long

c) 3.1 cm long d) None

Q10. The development of the mammary gland in male and females is similar upto;

a) Mammary Crest b) Mammary line

c) Mammary bud d) All the Above

Q11. In bovines the development of teats begins by about;

a) 20 d b) 30 d

c) 45 d d) 60 d

Q12. *Primary sprout,* a solid core of cells is formed when **age of** embryo is;

a) 20 d b) 40 d

c) 60 d d) 80d

Q13. Each teat has one teat pore to drain the milk in cows, buffaloes, sheep, goat, guinea pigs, rat **and** mice but horses has;

a) 2 pores b) 3 pores

c) 5 pores d) 7 pores

Q14. Secondary sprouts formation in mammary gland takes place at ;

a) 5-7 wks b) 9-13 wks
c) 13-14 wks d) 15-17 wks

Q15. Secondary Sprouts **in mammary gland** gives rise to ;

a) Gland cistern b) Major ducts
c) Teats cistern d) Teats canal

Q16. Canalization **in primary sprout** begins in bovine fetus when embryo is;

a) 13 cm long b) 15 cm long
c) 17 cm long d) 19 cm long.

Q17. Mammary growth form birth to puberty occurs at the same rate as general body growth and is referred as;

a) Isometric growth b) Allometric growth
c) Both a & b d) None

Q18. Allometric phase of growth **of mammary gland** take place at about 2-3 months;

a) Before puberty b) After puberty
c) From birth to puberty d) None

Q19. When the rate of mammary gland growth becomes faster (3.5 times) than the rest of the body, **it**is known as ;

a) Allometric phase of growth
b) Isometric phase of growth
c) Both a& b
d) None

Q20. Inruminants, **the** fundamental developmental unit in the mammary tissue is;

a) TDLU b) TEB
c) Both d) None

Q21. The growth of mammary gland is negligible during recurring estrous cycle **of cows** due to;

a) Asynchronous level of estrogen and progesterone

b) Synchronous level of estrogen and progesterone

c) Higher level of cortisol

d) None

Q22. MammaryVEGF-A, a multifunctionalcytokine which stimulates;

a) Angiogenesis,

b) Increases vascular permeability towater andproteins,

c) Causes vasodilatation and formation of fenestrationsin endothelial cells

d) All the above

Q23. Growth hormone can stimulate mammary growth at all stages of development through increased hepatic synthesis of the following factor;

a) IGF-1 b) EGF

c) TGF d) None

Q24. Placental lactogen (PL) have the characteristics of ;

a) Prolactin b) GH

c) Cortisol d) Both a and b

Q25. Which of the following does not have placental lactogen in circulation;

a) Rat &rabbit b) Mice& rabbit

c) Pig&rabbit d) Goat and rabbits

Q26. CBG binds with the following hormone;

a) Glucocorticoids b) GH

c) PRL d) T_4

Q27. Local production of following factor inhibits mammary growth during the pre-pubertal period and between estrous cycles;

a) TGF-α
b) TGF-β
c) EGF
d) All the above

Q28. The following growth factors stimulate mammary gland growth;

a) EGF
b) TGF-α
c) Both a & b
d) None

Q29. Mammary parenchyma tissue is positively correlated with following hormone;

a) GH
b) Prolactin
c) Cortisol
d) None

Q30. Recurring pregnancy and lactations result **increase**in milk production by about;

a) 10%
b) 20%
c) 30%
d) 40%

Q31. Hypophysectomy of pregnant cows results **in**;

a) Suppression of subsequent lactation
b) No effect on subsequent lactation
c) Increased MY in subsequent lactation
d) None

Q32. Injection of Prolactin in normal rats and mice results i**n**;

a) Initiation of lactation
b) Inhibition of lactation
c) Does not affect lactation
d) None

Q33. In rats, Prolactin hormone is;

a) Luteolytic
b) Luteotrophic
c) Both the above
d) None

Q34. Theperiparturient surge of the following hormone is essential for normal lactogenesis;

a) GH b) Cortisol

c) Prolactin d) Estrogen

Q35. Low levels of â lactoglobulin and casein are synthesized in the mammary cells during;

a) Last trimester of pregnancy

b) During II stage of lactogenesis

c) Both the above

d) None

Q36. During II-stage of lactogenesis,the copious secretion of milk occurs due to;

a) Synthesis of fat b) Synthesis of protein

c) Synthesis of lactose d) All the above

Q37. Mammary epithelial cells aquires the ability to synthesize and secrete milk constituents during the;

a) Galactopoiesis b) Mammogenesis

c) Lactogenesis d) Ductal morphogenesis

Q38. Stage I of lactogenesis is not associated with any one of the following;

a) Increased synthesis of enzymes

b) Formation of colostrums

c) Uptake of immunoglobulin's

d) Synthesis of á-lactalbumin.

Q39. The extracellular matrix components which are important for mammary growth and function are produced by;

a) Epithelial cell b) Stromal cell

c) Myoepithelial cell d) Both a and b

Q40. Cortisol hormone induces **the following in mammary gland of peripartuvient cows;**

a) Synthesis of protein
b) Differentiation of golgi apparatus
c) Differentiation of ER
d) All the above
e) None

Q41. During lactose synthesis the enzyme á-lactalbumin interacts with the **enzyme**galactosyl transferase in;

a) RER b) ER
c) Golgi apparatus d) None

Q42. The formation and update of immunoglobulins increases during;

a) Ist phase of lactogenesis b) IInd phase of lactogenesis
c) Day of parturition d) Both a and b

Q43. In pre-pubertal heifers the high feeding level reduces plasma level of;

a) PRL b) T4
c) Cortisol d) GH

Q44. Recent studies suggests that GH and IGF-I mediate ductal development togetherwith the following hormone;

a) Progesterone b) Estrogen
c) PRL d) All the above

Q45. During pregnancy higher levels of progesterone inhibits;

a) Upregulation of Prolactin b) Down regulation of Prolactin
c) Upregulation of GH d) None

Q46. Prepartum plasma progesterone concentration decline on day;

a) -8 to -7d b) -6 to -5d
c) -4 to -3d d) -2 to -1d

Q47. The TBG bind with the following hormone;

a) GH b) Thyroid hormone
c) Prolactin d) Glucocorticoids

Q48. The placental lactogen is not secreted by the placenta is;

a) Pigs b) Rabbits
c) Mice d) Both a and

Q49. Which prostaglandin in is most potent in terms of luteolytic action;

a) PGE1 b) PGE2
c) PGF1α d) PGF2α

Q50. The glucocorticoid level begins to rise by about;

a) 10 d prepartum b) 7 d prepartum
c) 4 d prepartum d) 1 d prepartum

Model Objective Type Questions II

Q1. In cattle the milking induced release of following hormone decreases with advancing stage of lactation;

a) Gluco**co**rticoids b) PRL
c) GH d) None

Q2. At high ambient temperature (>35°c), the higher **producing cows** secrete;

a) Higher quantities of glucocorticoids than low producers
b) Lower quantities of glucocorticoids than low producers
c) Similar quantities of glucocorticoids as for low Producers
d) None

Q3. Lactating mammary tissue in comparison to non lactating mammary tissue possesses;

a) 2 times more glucocorticoid receptors
b) 4 times more glucocorticoid receptors

c) 6times more glucocorticoid receptors

d) 8times more glucocorticoid receptors

Q4. Plasma concentration of the following hormone parallel very closely to the milk concentration in bovines;

a) GH b) Progesterone

c) Estrogen d) PRL

Q5. Neurophysin is a carrier protein for the hormone;

a) IGF-I b) PRL

c) Oxytocin d) Glucocorticoids

Q6. The excitatory neuron is the neuro- endocrine reflex are;

a) Nor-adrenergic neuron b) Adrenergic neuron

c) Cholinergic neuron d) None

Q7. During the synthesis, the oxytocin granules moves down the axon to the posterior pituitary gland at the rate of;

a) 1-2 mm/hr. b) 2-3 mm/hr.

c) 3-4 mm/hr. d) 4-5 mm/hr.

Q8. The storage depots for the neuro-secretory granules of oxytocin-neurophysin is;

a) Herring bodies b) Colostral bodies

c) Bodies of donn'e d) None

Q9. The contractile cell of the mammary gland is;

a) Epithelial cell b) Fibroblasts

c) Myoepithelial cell d) None

Q10. Sympathectomy results is;

a) Decreased rate of milk flow

b) Increased rate of milk flow

c) Increased or decreased milk flow rate

d) None

Q11. Release of catecholamine's decrease milk yield due to;

a) Increase tone of smooth muscle

b) Increase tone of blood vessel

c) Partial occlusion of mammary ducts

d) All the above

Q12. The primiparous cows may suffer from stress of milking in early postpartum period loading to inhibition of oxytocin release from ant. Pituitary gland and is referred as;

a) Central inhibition b) Peripheral inhibition

c) Both a and b d) None

Q13. The hormone which causes let down of milk is known as;

a) GH b) Glucocorticoids

c) Vasopressin d) Oxytocin

Q14. The prepartum surge of Prolactin is related to;

a) Normal secretion of milk

b) Copious secretion of milk

c) No effect on milk secretion

d) Both a and b

Q15. Administration of ergot drugs leads to suppression of plasma level of;

a) GH b) Cortisol

c) IGF-I d) PRL

Q16. Prolactin hormone binds with the receptors located in;

a) Cell surface b) Cytoplasm

c) Nucleus d) None of above

Q17. The lactogenic effects of Prolactin and cortisol are mediated by;

a) Decrease in intracellular concentration

b) Increase in intracellular cAMP concentration

c) No change in cAMP concentration
d) None

Q18. Injection of progesterone during pregnancy result in;

a) On set of lactogenesis b) Inhibition of lactogenesis
c) No effect on lactogenesis d) Abortion

Q19. Which hormone has binding affinity with glucocorticoids receptors in the cytoplasm;

a) PRL b) GH
c) Estrogen d) Progesterone

Q20. A combination of the following hormone induces lactation in repeate breeder/dry animals;

a) Estrogen and GH
b) Progesterone and Prolactin
c) Estrogen and progesterone
d) GH and Prolactin

Q21. Prepartum milking of cows generally initiates lactation in pregnant animals due to;

a) Inhibition of PIF secretion
b) Stimulation of CRF release
c) Stimulation of release of GH
d) Both a and b

Q22. Administration of TRH stimulates milk yield in cattle and women due to;

a) Secretion of GH b) Secretion of PRL
c) Secretion of cortisol d) Both a and b

Q23. Administration ofGH does not affect production of milk in the following;

a) Cattle b) Buffalo
c) Rat d) Goat

Q24. Increasing concentration of dopamine inhibits milking induced release of the following hormone;

a) GH b) PRL

c) IGF-I d) Glucocorticoids

Q25. Suppression of Prolactin by ergot drugs inhibits lactation performance in;

a) Monogastric species b) Ruminat species

c) Both a and b d) None

Q26. Sergical removal of thyroid gland result is;

a) No change in milk yield b) Increase in milk yield

c) Decrease in milk yield d) None

Q27. The major growth of mammary gland takes place during;

a) Lactation b) Dry state

c) Pregnancy d) Puberty

Q28. Hematoxylein stain is used to reveal the extent of development of;

a) Ductal growth is mammary fat pad

b) Lobule-alveolar growth in fat pad

c) Both a and b

d) None

Q29. In mare, the pregnant mare serum gonadotropin (PMSG) disappears **in the blood**after;

a) 100 d of gestation b) 125 d of gestation

c) 150 d of gestation d) None

Q30. Human chorionic gonadotropin (HCG) appears in the blood and urine of pregnant human approximately;

a) 16 days after ovulation b) 20 days after ovulation

c) 24 days after ovulation d) none

Q31. HCG disappears from blood and urine at approximately;

a) 120 d of gestation
b) 140 d of gestation
c) 160 d of gestation
d) 180 d of gestation

Q32. Placental lactogen is a;

a) Protein hormone
b) Glycoprotein hormone
c) Protein hormone without a CHO component
d) None

Q33. The amount of milk produced by the mammary gland is dependent on;

a) No. of epithelial cell
b) Precursor supplied to MG
c) Supply of MG to hormone
d) Frequent removal of milk
e) All the above

Q34. The cows have mammary gland in the inguinal region which is;

a) 1 in number
b) 2 in number
c) 4 in number
d) None

Model Objective Type Questions III

Q1. In sow, the mammary glands are located in;

a) Inguinal region
b) Thorax
c) Abdomen
d) None

Q2. In elephants, the mammary glands are located in;

a) Abdomen
b) Thorax
c) Inguinal
d) All the above

Q3. Rat mammary glands are located in the following regions;

a) Thorax
b) Inguinal
c) Abdomen
d) All the above

Q4. In cows the rear quarter of mammary gland are;

a) Larger than fore quarter b) Shorter than fore quarter
c) Similar in nature d) None

Q5. The cows may have more than four teats, which are referred as ;

a) Supernumerary teats b) Extra teats
c) Accessory teats d) All the above

Q6. The lateral suspensory ligaments of mammary glands are;

a) Fibrous and elastic
b) Fibrous and non-elastic
c) arise from subpubic/prepubic tendons
d) Both b and c

Q7. The blood leaves udder of a cow by the following routes;

a) external pudic vein
b) subcutaneous abdominal veen
c) Both a and b
d) Venous circle

Q8. The lactating mammary gland **receives**;

a) 5 % of cardiac output b) 8 % of cardiac output
c) 10 % of cardiac output d) 12 % of cardiac output

Q9. The ratio of blood though the udder to milk yield is about;

a) 1000:1 ml b) 800:1 ml
c) 600:1 ml d) 500:1 ml

Q10. Lymph composition is similar to the blood plasma except that lymph has about;

a) ¼ protein content of plasma
b) ½ protein content of plasma
c) 1/6 protein content of plasma
d) None

Q11. Rabbit has following number of streak canal /teat;

a) 1-2 b) 3-4
c) 5-6 d) 10-12

Q12. The mammary gland lack streak canal in the following;

a) Rat and Dog b) Rabbit and Dog
c) Women and Dog d) Women and rat

Q13. A group of alveoli and their associated ducts in mammary gland constitute ;

a) Lobule b) Lobe
c) Both a and b d) None

Q14. which of the following structure have single layered epithelium lining;

a) Terminal ducts b) Larger ducts
c) Alveoli d) Terminal ducts and alveoli

Q15. In ruminants, secretion of milk is;

a) Phasic process b) Interminant process
c) Continuous process d) None

Q16. The maintenance of established lactation is referred as;

a) Lactogenesis b) Mammogenesis
c) Biosynthesis d) Galactopoiesis

Q17. **In cows, the** maintenance of lactation depends on;

a) Synthesis of milk
b) Removal of milk
c) Action of galactopoietic hormones
d) All the above

Q18. The standard length of lactation in goat is;

a) 300 days b) 250 days
c) 200 days d) 150 days

Q19. The programmed death of the mammary epithelial cells is known as;

a) Meiosis
b) Mitosis
c) Apoptosis
d) Morphogenesis

Q20. Milk production during lactation can be maintained by maintaining the;

a) No.'s of alveoli cell
b) Synthetic activity/mammary cell
c) Efficiency of milk ejection reflex
d) All the above

Q21. Administration of L-DOPA **in** non-ruminants results in;

a) Reduced milk yield
b) Inhibition of milk ejection
c) Both a and b
d) No effect on a and b above

Q22. The minimum requirement in lypox.rat to restore lactation is;

a) PRL alone
b) PRL + glucocorticoids
c) PRL + glucocorticoids + GH
d) None

Q23. Administration of TRH stimulate secretion of following hormones in cattle;

a) PRL
b) GH
c) Thyroxine
d) All the above

Q24. IGF_I is a single chain peptide **hormone** and have;

a) 50 aa
b) 60 aa
c) 70 aa
d) 80 aa

Q25. The available literature suggest that IGF-I is resistant to;

a) Milk boiling
b) Pasteurization
c) Both
d) None

Q26. The molecular weight of GH is;

a) 26000 b) 36000

c) 46000 d) 56000

Q27. The mature form of bGH is a single-chain polypeptide containing following amino acids;

a) 141 b) 161

c) 181 d) 191

Q28. The homology between bovine and ovine GH is;

a) 97% b) 67%

c) 57% d) 47%

Q29. An arterial infusion of IGF-I into the mammary gland stimulates;

a) Blood flow to MG b) Increase in milk production

c) Both a and b d) None

Q30. In laboratory animal, the adrenalectomy will lead to;

a) Reduce enzymatic function

b) Reduce casein in RNA synthesis

c) Impair milk secretion

d) All the above

Q31. One of the following operation steps lactation completely;

a) Adrenectomy b) Ovariectomy

c) Hypophyectomy d) All the above

Q32. The suckling induced release of glucocorticoids decline with advancement of lactation in;

a) Cows b) Buffaloes

c) Rat d) Goat

Q33. At high ambient temperature (>35°C)the secretion of glucocorticoids in high producing cows;

a) Decreases b) Increases

c) Remain same d) None

Model Objective Type Questions IV

Q1. Feeding of thyroprotein in cattle results in;

a) Increase in milk yield b) Decrease in milk yield

c) Milk yield remain same d) None

Q2. The thyroxine hormone binds with the following globulin;

a) CBG b) TBG

c) Neurophysin d) None

Q3. Thyroid stimulating hormone is secreted by;

a) Hypothalamus b) Posterior pituitary gland

c) Anterior pituitary gland d) Thyroid gland

Q4. The major biologically active form of thyroid hormone is;

a) T_4 b) T_3

c) T_2 d) None

Q5. Mammary gland of rat has;

a) Type I deiodinase activity

b) Type II deiodinase activity

c) Type III deiodinase activity

d) None

Q6. Mammary gland of Sow has;

a) Type III deiodinase enzyme

b) Type II deiodinase enzyme

c) Type I deiodinase enzyme

d) Both b and c

Q7. The mammary type II deiodinase enzyme is present in the mammary gland of;

a) Rat b) Mouse

c) Cows d) Both b and c

Q8. During lactation, the high activity of deiodinase enzyme in the mammary gland of cows results in more local production of following hormone;

a) T4 b) T2

c) T3 d) All the above

Q9. Mammary gland has been found to synthesize following hormones;

a) GH and Prolactin b) Leptin

c) PTHrP d) All the above

Q10. The **low** levels of leptin in lactating rats possibly contribute to;

a) Hypophagia b) Hyperphagia

c) No change in feed intakes d) None

Q11. The PTHrP is expressed during lactation and is secreated by;

a) Epithelial cell b) Myoepithelial cell

c) Stromal cell d) none

Q12. The oxytocin binding sites are located on;

a) Epithelial cell b) Stromal cell

c) Myoepithelial cell d) None

Q13. During lactation the receptors for the following hormone are virtually absent in mammary gland;

a) Estrogen b) Progesterone

c) Prolactin d) GH

Q14. The involution of Mammary gland during the dry period is accelerated by the injection of hormone;

a) Progesterone b) Prolactin

c) Estrogen d) IGF-I

Q15. The udder weight and udder capacity of cows increases up to;

a) 6-8 yrs of age b) 8-10 yrs of age
c) 4-6 yrs of age d) None

Q16. After the parturition the mammary growth does not occur in the following;

a) Cow b) Goat
c) Buffalo d) Sheep

Q17. One of the following is more resistant to the process of involution;

a) Mammary DNA b) Hydroxyproline
c) Cell numbers d) None

Q18. Placental lactogen are not present in;

a) Sheep b) Goat
c) Cow d) Rat

Q19. Suckling decrease release of the following;

a) PRL b) PIF
c) TRH d) GnRH

Q20. Suckling causes release of following hormone in ruminants;

a) Prolactin b) GH
c) Cortisol d) Both a and c

Q21. Each mammary epithelial cell contains following number of binding sites for cortisol hormone;

a) 5500 b) 6500
c) 7500 d) 8500

Q22. Hypocalcemia at parturition is associated with;

a) Rise in PTH hormone b) Decrease in plasma ca++
c) Both a and b d) None

Q23. Pineal gland contains following biogenic amines;

a) Melatonin b) Serotonin
c) Catecholamines d) All the above

Q24. Lactose synthesis takes place in the;

a) ER b) Golgi
c) Cytoplasm d) None

Q25. Which of the following act as a scavenger to solubilize the dyeing cells;

a) Lysosomes b) Mitochondria
c) Golgi apparatus d) ER

Q26. The structure that does not allow free passage of substances between epithelial cells are known as;

a) Tight junctions b) Myoepithelial cells
c) Bodies of donn'c d) None

Q27. The secretion of mammary gland which involve complete loss of entire cell to form the secretory product is called as;

a) Apocrine b) Merocrine
c) Holocrine d) None

Q28. The release of fat from the epithelial cell occurs by the process of;

a) Apocrine b) Merocrine
c) Endocrine d) Holocrine

Model Objective Type Questions V

Q1. The decline in milk yield in unit time is a constant percentage of the previous production and is referred as;

a) Involution b) Persistency
c) Galactopoiesis d) None

Q2. Complete mammary denervation in sheep and goat results in;

a) No effect on milk yield
b) No effect on milk ejection
c) No effect on milk production
d) All the above

Q3. Intact somatic sensory innervations of the mammary gland are necessary for milk production in;

a) Sheep b) Goat
c) Rat d) Cat

Q4. The ribosomal particle is the site of synthesis of;

a) Fat b) Lactose
c) Protein d) Glucose

Q5. Membranes of the mammary gland is made up of;

a) 50-60% protein b) 40-50% lipid
c) 40-50% protein d) Both a and b

Q6. Basal part of the epithelial cell of mammary gland has many irregular placed "feet", which;

a) Increase surface area of cell
b) Increase up the efficiency of cell
c) Both a and b
d) None

Q7. During the intracellular phase of secretion of milk there is a progressive;

a) Distension of the alveoli
b) Reduction of the alveoli
c) Neither distend nor reduce in size
d) All the above

Q8. During active intracellular secretion ,the epithelial cell of mammary gland are;

a) Small and columnar b) Tall and columnar
c) Flattened and small d) None

Q9. Milk protein and lactose are extruded via secretory vesicles by the process of;

a) Exocytosis b) Reverse pinocytosis
c) Pinching off d) None

Q10. The fat laden cells of the colostrum are known as;

a) Bodies of donn'e b) Desquamated cells
c) Histiocytes d) None

Q11. Milk and blood have the same osmotic pressure of;

a) 4.4 atmosphere b) 5.5atmosphere
c) 6.6 atmosphere d) 7.7 atmosphere

Q12. Lactose in milk account for about;

a) 80% atmospheric pressure
b) 70%atmospheric pressure
c) 60% atmospheric pressure
d) 50% atmospheric pressure

Q13. Casein of milk is bound in the milk with;

a) Phosphorus b) Magnesium
c) Sodium d) Calcium

Q14. One of the following is a non-essential amino acid in milk proteins;

a) Methionine b) Lysine
c) Glutamine d) Valine

Q15. Thee is no mammary uptake of amino acids in;

a) Lactating mammary gland
b) Virgin mammary gland
c) Dry mammary gland
d) None

Q16 .Caseen is secreted into milk in the form of;

a) Secretory vesicles b) Micelle
c) Droplets d) None

Q17. The following percentage of total milk calcium binds with the casein micelles;

a) 50% b) 70%
c) 90% d) 100%

Q18. The lactating mammary gland of goat derives 30-50% of its energy from the oxidation of glucose and the following percentage from blood acetate;

a) 10-20% b) 20-30%

c) 30-40% d) 40-50%

Q19. Of the total blood caloric the following percentage of calorie is transferred to milk by the mammary gland;

a) Nearly 80% b) Nearly 70%

c) Nearly 60% d) Nearly 50%

Q20. The infusion of acetate in mammary gland of goats leads to;

a) Increase in milk yield b) No change in milk yield

c) Decrease in milk yield d) None

Q21. Infusion of glucose into mammary gland of goat results in;

a) 62% increase in milk yield

b) 87% increase in lactose

c) No effect on fat percentage

d) All the above

Q22. The major source of blood glucose in ruminants is;

a) Acetate b) Butyrate

c) Propionate d) Valerate

Q23. Source of blood glucose in non-ruminants is;

a) Gluconeogenesis b) Absorption from gut

c) Both a and b d) None

Q24. lactose,a milk sugar contains;

a) 1mol.glucose+1 mol.galactose

b) 1mol.glucose+1 mol. Lactose

c) 2mol.glucose+2 mol.galactose

d) None

Q25. The lactose synthetase enzyme is made up of;

a) Galactosyl transferase b) α-lactalbumin
c) β-lactoglobulin d) Both a and b

Q26. Lactose is secreted along with the following enzymes via the golgi;

a) β-lactoglobulin b) α-lactalbumin
c) Both a and b d) None

Q27. Galactosaemia is a decrease of human in which following cannot be utilized;

a) Glucose b) Lactose
c) Galactose d) None

Q28. Galactosaemia patient lacks the following enzyme;

a) Lactose-1- phosphate uridyl transferase
b) Galactose-1-phosphate uridyl transferase
c) Glucose-1- phosphate uridyl transferase
d) None

Q29. Lactose intolerance in human being is due to lack of following enzyme;

a) Amylase b) Lactase
c) Kinase d) Acetyl COA carboxylase

Q30. Milk fat contains large proportions of;

a) Short chain FAs b) Long chain FAs
c) Both a and b d) None

Q31. The depot fat of ruminant is very high in;

a) Palmitic acid b) Stearic acid
c) Lactic acid d) None

Q.32. The average milk cow secretes about twice as much fat as in milk due to;

a) Dietry effect b) Denovo synthesis
c) Mobilization of reserves d) None

Q33. Milk fat contains;

a) 70% triglycerides b) 80% triglycerides
c) 90% triglycerides d) 98% triglycerides

Q34. Which type of fatty acids is synthesized by the mammary gland?

a) Long chain b) Short chain
c) Both a and b d) None

Q35. The mammary gland of a cow does not utilize the following for milk fat synthesis;

a) Phospholipids b) Cholesterol esters
c) Free cholesterol d) All the above

Q36. During fat synthesis, the enzyme which convert stearic acid to oleic acid in the mammary gland is;

a) Desaturase b) Synthetase
c) Carboxylase d) None

Q37. Synthesis of short chained fatty acid in mammary tissue of ruminants and non-ruminant occurs is;

a) Golgi apparatus b) Cytosol
c) RER d) None

Q38. Acyl carrier protein (ACP) is a carrier of;

a) Amino acids intermediates
b) Fatty acids intermediates
c) Intermediates lactose synthesis
d) None

Q39. The milk flow from alveoli to cisternal space is;

a) Continuous b) Rhythemic
c) Both a and b d) None

Q40. About 70% of the mammary gland by volume is;

a) Parenchyma b) Non parenchyma
c) Lumen d) None

Model Objective Type Questions VI

Q1. In ruminants, the acetate entering the mammary gland participates in;

a) Energy production b) Fatty acid synthesis
c) Both a and b d) None

Q2. Denovo synthesis of fatty acid by the ruminant mammary gland involves fatty acid of;

a) C4-C16 b) $\geq$ C16
c) Both and b d) None

Q3. In ruminants, the regulatory enzyme in milk fat synthesis is;

a) Malonyl COA-ACP transferase
b) β-ketoayl reductase
c) Enoyl reductase
d) Acetyl COA carboxylase

Q4. BHBA taken up by ruminant mammary gland is used primararly in;

a) Fatty acid synthesis b) Energy production
c) Both and b d) None

Q5. First reaction of the fatty acid synthesis in mammary gland is catalyzed by enzyme;

a) Fatty acid synthetase b) Acetyl CoA carboxylase
c) Reductase d) Fatty acyl deacylase

Q6. The marker of onset of lactogenesis during periparturient period is;

a) Calcium b) Citrate
c) Immunoglobulins d) None

Q7. In cows,cold stress increases plasma hormone levels of;

a) Thyroxine b) Glucocorticoids
c) Calcitonin d) Both a and b

Q8. Cattle have higher plasma Prolactin in summer due to;

a) Heat stress
b) More water metabolism
c) More electrolyte metabolism
d) All the above

Q9. Animals that secrete more potassium in sweat display reduced plasma concentration of;

a) ADH b) PRL
c) Aldosterone d) None

Q10. The pH of ruminant milk in comparison to plasma is;

a) Higher b) Lower
c) Similar d) None

Q11. The elevation of plasma ketone bodies during pregnancy in cows is known as;

a) Ketosis b) Metabolic acidosis
c) Toxemia d) None

Q12. Ketosis in animals leads to;

a) Increased plasma ketone bodies
b) Higher FFAs in plasma
c) Low cholesterol levels
d) All the above

Q13. Milk fever a metabolic disease occurs in cows when plasma calcium level decrease to;

a) < 10 mg% b) <8 mg%
c) <5 mg% d) <3 mg%

Q14. The low milk fat syndrome in cows occur when dietary fiber is less than;

a) 10-12% b) 12-14%
c) 15-17% d) 17-19%

Q15. Cows calving during cooler months produce more milk and have;

a) More milk fat b) More SNF
c) Both a and b d) None

Q16. The maintenance requirement of cattle increases during;

a) Heat stress b) Cold stress
c) Both a and b d) None

Q17. The primary reason for the greater heat tolerance of indicus than Boss Taurus cattle is due to;

a) Lower milk yield b) Low feed intake
c) Low BMR d) All the above

Q18. Following animals do not pant;

a) Rat and Horse b) Cow
c) Buffalo d) None

Q19. Panting in animals result in;

a) Less removal of blood CO2
b) Respiratory alkalosis
c) Decrease in blood Ph
d) None

Q20. The feeding of more concentrate and less roughage during summer to the cows leads to change in ratio of;

a) Propionate to butyrate b) Acetate to butyrate
c) Acetate to propionate d) None

Q21. Lactating cows sweat contains high concentration of;

a) Sodium b) potassium
c) Magnesium d) None

Q22. lactoferrin concentration in the dry bovine mammary gland is;

a) Lower b) Higher
c) Normal d) None

Q23. Enzyme xanthive oxidase,is a major component of;

a) Secretary vesicle b) Fat globule
c) Protein structure d) None

Q24. The predominant Ig found in the bovine milk and colostrum is;

a) IgA b) IgE
c) IgM d) IgG

Q25. Milk contains;

a) High Na and low K+ b) High Na and high K+
c) Low Na and high K+ d) None

Q26. One gram of active mammary secretary tissue can secrete about;

a) 0-1g milk/d b) 1-2 g milk/d
c) 2-3 g milk/d d) 3-4 g milk/d

Q27. Most abundant lipid in milk fat is;

a) Monoglycerides b) Diglycerides
c) Triglycerides d) Cholesterol esters

Q28. Residual milk is the amount of milk that is left in the udder after milking and contains;

a) High fat b) Low fat
c) High protein d) Low protein

Q29. The milk fat supplies energy as much as;

a) 100 Kcal/100 g milk b) 300Kcal/100 g milk
c) 500 Kcal/100 g milk d) 700Kcal/100g milks

Q30. Milk of very high fat contents is characteristic of artic and aquatic species as young ones require;

a) Less energy b) More energy
c) More fat for insulation d) Both b and c

Q31. Cows colostrums contain;

a) More fat less lactose
b) More minerals and protein
c) Less fat and less lactose
d) Both a and b

Model Objective Type Questions VII

Q1. Kangaroos produces milk fat devoid of;

a) Long chain fatty acids
b) Short chain fatty acids
c) Medium chain fatty acids
d) None

Q2. In general cows which have large diameter of teat have;

a) Faster milk flow
b) Prone to mastitis
c) Both a and b
d) None

Q3. Frustenbrg's rosette is located at the junction of;

a) Teat eastern and gland cistern
b) Teat cistern and teat canal
c) Teat canal and teat pore
d) None

Q4. Machine striping of teats at the end of machine milking involves;

a) Pulling the milking cluster after milking
b) Pulling the milking cluster at the fag end of milking
c) Pulling down milking cluster with simultaneous hand message of udder
d) Pulling down milking cluster without hand message of udder

Q5. The incomplete milking is associated with;

a) Reduced milk yield
b) Reduced persistancy
c) Increased mastitis
d) All the above

Q6. The cholesterol content in bovine milk is;

a) 0.1-0.2%
b) 0.2-0.3%
c) 0.3-0.4%
d) 0.4-0.5%

Q7. The milk of seal contains;

a) High lactose
b) Low lactose
c) No lactose
d) None

Q8. The iron- binding protein of milk is;

a) Transferrin
b) Lactoferrin
c) á-lactalbulin
d) Both a and b

Q9. In terms of electrical resistance, the cows are following times more susceptible to shock than humans;

a) 5 times
b) 10 times
c) 20 times
d) 25 times

Q10. The cows milk production is rarely affected until exposure to;

a) 1 milliamps
b) 3 milliamps
c) 5 milliamps
d) 7 milliamps

Q11. Studies has shown that during lactation, the leucocytes probably do not enter the milk space rapidly until;

a) One of secretory cells dies
b) Secretory cell slough off membrane
c) Both a and b
d) None

Q12. The milk SCC measurement could be used to indicate;

a) Inflammation of udder
b) Loss of milk yield due to mastitis
c) Quality of milk
d) All the above

Q13. The average normal milk SCC in a healthy udder is;

a) 1.0lakh cells/ml
b) 2.0 lakh cells/ml
c) 3.0 lakh cells/ml
d) 4.0 lakh cells/ml

Q14. Extending the milking period in lactation cows decrease average secretion rate after period of;

a) 5 hr b) 10 hr
c) 20 hr d) 30 hr

Q15. In a cow which has not been milked, the milk secretion stops after;

a) 20 hr b) 25 hr
c) 30 hr d) 35 hr

Q16. Within one hour of last milking the residual milk moves into cistern from alveoli and small ducts and the udder pressure increase by approximately;

a) 4 mm Hg b) 8 mm Hg
c) 12 mm Hg d) 16 mm Hg

Q17. The mineral in milk that can be altered appreciably are;

a) Iodine b) Iron
c) Both d) None

Q18. While milking the cows, approximately following percentage of milk is not removed by normal milking;

a) 1-10% b) 10-20%
c) 15-25% d) 20-30%

Q19. During milking, the peak milk flow rates occurs between;

a) 1-2 min. after start of milking
b) 1.5-2.5 min. after start of milking
c) 2.0-3.0 min. after start of milking
d) 2.5-3.5 min. after start of milking

Q20. Electrical stimulation of the hypothalamus leads to release of oxytocin which is;

a) More than the hand milking associated release of oxytocin
b) More than the milking stimulates

c) Similar to hand induced release of oxytocin
d) Less than hand induced release of oxytocin

Q21. In anesthetized goats ,the milk ejection reflex is usually;

a) Excited b) Inhibited
c) Normal d) None

Q22. The conditioned release of oxytocin in a cow occurs due to;

a) Auditory stimuli of milking
b) Visual stimuli of milking
c) Sight of milking parlor
d) All the above

Q23. Frequent milking of a cow from twice a day to 3 times a day result in;

a) Decrease milk yield b) Increase milk yield
c) No change in milk yield d) none

Q24. Physiological factors that contribute to increased milk yield are;

a) Less intra- mammary pressure
b) Higher hormone levels galactopoietics
c) Less FIL conc.
d) All the above

Q25. Nearly one-fifth of new intra- mammary infection occurs during the first;

a) 1-2 wk of dry period b) 2-3wk of dry period
c) 3-4wk of dry period d) None

Q26. The dry cow therapy drugs should remain active in the udder for the following period to effectively check intra-mammary injections;

a) 1-2 wk b) 2-3wk
c) 3-4 wk d) 4-5 wk

Q27. The cell mediated immune response is mediated by;

a) T-lymphocytes b) B-lymphocytes

c) Both a and b d) None

Q28. The major classes (isotypes) of immunoglobulin's are;

a) 2 types b) 3 types

c) 4 types d) 5 types

Q29. The basic structure of all the Ig (immunoglobulin) has;

a) 2 chains b) 3 chains

c) 4 chains d) 5 chains

Q30. In mammary gland of a cow, the IgA is synthesized by;

a) Epithelial cells b) Plasma cells

c) Stroma cell d) None

Q31. When a lactating cow is exposed to an antigen for the first time, the synthesis of IgM antibodies exceeds than that of;

a) IgG b) IgA

c) IgE d) Igd

Q32. The external pudic vein of mammary gland arise from;

a) Cranial branch of vein b) Caudal branch of vein

c) Both a and b d) none

Q33.In the perinral vein of mammary gland, the direction of blood flow is;

a) Away from the udder b) Towards the udder

c) Both a and b d) None

Q34. In the virgin sheep, goat and cows the following vein carries all the venous blood back to the heart;

a) External pudic vein

b) Subcutaneous abdomen vein

c) Perineal vein

d) none

Q35. Subuctaneous abdominal vein is also known as;

a) Perineal vein b) Milk vein
c) External pudic vein d) None

Q36. During the lying state the venous blood leaves the udder through;

a) Subcutaneous abdomen vein
b) External pudic vein
c) Perineal vein
d) None

Q37. Rear quarters of udder are usually larger than the forequarters and produces about;

a) 50% of total milk b) 60% of total milk
c) 70%of total milk d) None

Q38. The following ligaments provides support and absorbs shocks created when cow is walking or lying down;

a) Lateral suspensory ligaments
b) Median suspensory ligaments
c) Both a and b
d) None

Q39. The sympathetic innervations to the mammary gland are;

a) Adrenergic b) Cholinergic
c) Both a and b d) None

Q40. The ratio of capillaries to lymph vessel in mammary gland is;

a) 25:1 b) 50:1
c) 100:1 d) 150:1

Q41. Myoepithelial cells takes about following time to fully contract;

a) 2 seconds b) 4 seconds
c) 6 seconds d) None

Q42. The time taken for transmission of teat stimulus to hypothalamus, release of oxytocin and reaching of oxytocin to heart and than myoepithelial cells is about;

a) 11-14 seconds b) 14-17 seconds

c) 17-19 seconds d) 19-22 seconds

Q43. In Rodents,the primary glucocorticoid is;

a) Cortisol b) Corticosterone

c) Both a and b d) None

Q44. The primary glucocorticoid cortisol is not related to;

a) Rodent b) Human

c) Cows d) Pigs

Answer Key

Model objective type question-I

Q1.c Q2.d Q3.b Q4.c Q5.d Q6.c Q7.c Q8.a Q9.b Q10.c

Q11.d Q12.d Q13.a Q14.c Q15.b Q16.d Q17.a Q18.a Q19.a Q20.a

Q21.a Q22.d Q23.a Q24.d Q25.c Q26.a Q27.b Q28.c Q29.a Q30.c

Q31.a Q32.c Q33.b Q34.c Q35.a Q36.c Q37.c Q38.d Q39.d Q40.d

Q41.a Q42.a Q43.d Q44.b Q45.a Q46.d Q47.b Q48.d Q49.d Q50.b

Model objective type question-II

Q1.b Q2.b Q3.b Q4.b Q5.c Q6.c Q7.b Q8.a Q9.c Q10.b

Q11.d Q12.a Q13.d Q14.b Q15.d Q16.a Q17.a Q18.b Q19.d Q20.c

Q21.d Q22.d Q23.c Q24.b Q25.a Q26.c Q27.c Q28.b Q29. Q30.a

Q31.c Q32.c Q33.e Q34.c

Model objective type question-III

Q1.c Q2.b Q3.d Q4.a Q5.d Q6.d Q7.c Q8.b Q9.d Q10.b

Q11.c Q12.c Q13.a Q14.d Q15.c Q16.d Q17.d Q18.d Q19.c Q20.d

Q21.c Q22.c Q23.d Q24.c Q25.b Q26.c Q27.d Q28.a Q29.c Q30.d

Q31.d Q32.c Q33.a

Model objective type question-IV

Q1.a Q2.b Q3.c Q4.b Q5.a Q6.d Q7.d Q8.c Q9.d Q10.b
Q11.a Q12.c Q13.b Q14.c Q15.a Q16.d Q17.b Q18.c Q19.b Q20.d
Q21.c Q22.c Q23.d Q24.b Q25.a Q26.a Q27.c Q28.d

Model objective type question-V

Q1.b Q2.d Q3.d Q4.c Q5.d Q6.c Q7.b Q8.b Q9.b Q10.a
Q11.c Q12.d Q13.d Q14.c Q15.c Q16.b Q17.c Q18.b Q19.a Q20.b
Q21.d Q22.c Q23.c Q24.a Q25.d Q26.b Q27.c Q28.b Q29.b Q30.a
Q31.b Q32.b Q33.d Q34.b Q35.d Q36.a Q37.b Q38.b Q39.b Q40.c

Model objective type question-VI

Q1.c Q2.a Q3.d Q4.a Q5.b Q6.b Q7.d Q8.d Q9.c Q10.b
Q11.c Q12.d Q13.c Q14.c Q15.c Q16.c Q17.d Q18.a Q19.b Q20.c
Q21.b Q22.b Q23.b Q24.d Q25.c Q26.b Q27.c Q28.a Q29.c Q30.d
Q31.d

Model objective type question-VII

Q1.b Q2.c Q3.b Q4.c Q5.d Q6.c Q7.c Q8.d Q9.b Q10.c
Q11.c Q12.d Q13.a Q14.a Q15.d Q16.b Q17.c Q18.c Q19.b Q20.a
Q21.b Q22.d Q23.b Q24.d Q25.a Q26.c Q27.c Q28.d Q29.c Q30.b
Q31.a Q32.c Q33.b Q34.a Q35.b Q36.b Q37.b Q38.b Q39.a Q40.c
Q41.c Q42.d Q43.b Q44.a

❑❑❑

Bibliography

Achmadi, J.; Yanagisawa, T.; Sano, H.; Terashima, Y., 1993. *Domest. Anim. Endocrinol.*, 10: 279-287.

Aggarwal, A.; *Mahendra Singh., 2005. Egyptian Journal of Dairy Sciences,* 32(1): 175-186.

Aggarwal, A.; Mahendra Singh., 2006. *Indian Dairyman,* 58(3): 49-59.

Aggarwal, A.; Mahendra Singh., 2007. *Ind. J. Agric. Economics,* 62: 272-279.

Aggarwal, A.; Mahendra Singh., 2009. *Indian J. Dairy Sci.,* 62(1): 35-38.

Aggarwal, A.; Mahendra Singh; Chopra, R.C., 2008. *Indian J. Dairy Sci.,* 61(1): 88-89.

Aggarwal. A.; Mahendra Singh., 2005. *Indian Journal of Dairy Sciences,* 58(4): 269-274.

Aggarwal. A.; Mahendra Singh., 2008. *Tropical Animal Health and Production,* 40(3): 223-228.

Ahima, R.S.; Flier, J.S., 2000. *Annu. Rev. Physiol.,* 62: 413-437.

Akers, R.M., 1985. *Dairy Sci.,* 68(2): 501-519.

Akers, R.M., 1990. Lactation physiology: a ruminant perspective. *Protoplasma,* 159: 96-111.

Akhtar, M.S.; Lodhi, L.A.; Farooq, A.A.; Ayaz, M.M.; Hussain, M. *et. al.,* 2012. *Pakistan Veterinary Journal,* 32(3): 435-437.

Amit Kumar; Avtar Singh, 2006. *Indian j. Anim. Res.,* 40(2): 95-100.

Ananth, C.; Gopalkrishnakone, P.; Kaur, C., 2003. *Hippocampus,* 13: 375-387.

Andersen, J.B.; Friggens, N.C.; Larse, T.; Vestergaard, M.; Ingvartsen, K.L., 2004. *J. Vety. Med.,* 51: 52-57.

Annen, E.L.; Collier, R.J.; McGuire, M. A.; Vicin, J.L., 2004. *J. Dairy Sci.,* 87: (E Suppl.): E66–E76.

Argherie, D., 2008. *Lucrari Scientific Med Vet Timisoara,* 12: 504-509.

Armstrong, D.V., 1994. *J. Dairy Sci.,* 77: 2044-2050. Berman, A. 2005. *J. Anim. Sci.,* 83: 1377-1384. Berman, A.; Folman, Y.; Kaim, M.; Mamen, M.; Herz, Z.; Wolfenson, D.; Arieli, A.; Graber. Y., 1985. *J. Dairy Sci.,* 68: 1488-1495. Borderas, T.F.; Pawluczuk, B.; de Passille, A. M.; Rushen. J., 2004. *J. Dairy Sci.,* 87: 2085-2093.

Ashutosh, M.; Singh, M., 2007. *Indian Journal of Dairy Science,* 60(6): 417-421.

Ashutosh, M.; Singh, M., 2008. *Indian Veterinary Journal,* 85(11): 1230-1231.

Ashwell, J.D.; Lu, F.W.M.; Vacchio, M.S., 2000. *Annual review of immunology,* 18: 309-345.

Auldist, M.J.; Coats, S.; Rogers, G.L.; McDowell, G.H., 1995. *Australian Journal of Experimental Agriculture,* 35(4): 427-436.

Auldist, M.J.; Prosser, C.G,. 1998. *Proceedings of the New Zealand Society of Animal Production,* 58: 41-43.

Bachman, K.C.; Wilford, D.H.; Head, H.H.; Wilcox, C.J.; Mahendra Singh., 1992. *J. Dairy Sci.,* 75: 1883-1890.

Baile, D.A; Buonomo, F.C., 1987. *J. Dairy Sci.,* 70: 467-473.

Baldwin, B.R.; Forsberg, NeE.; Hu, C.Y., 1985. *J. Dairy Sci.,* 68: 3394-3402.

Bass, E., J. Shani, Y. Givant, R. Yagil, and F.G. Sulman. 1974. Arch. Int. Pharmacodynami. Ther. 211: 188-192.

Bauer, M.E.; Perks, P.; Lightman, S.L.; Shanks, N.; 2001. *Physiology and Behavior,* 73(4): 525-532.

Bauman, D.E.; Currie, W.B.; Baldwin, R.L.; Plucinski, T., 1977. *Reproduction in Domestic Animals,* pp. 369.

Bauman, D.E.; Vernon, R.G., 1983. *Annual Review of Nutrition,* 13: 437-461 (DOI: 10.1146/annurev.nu. 13.070193.002253).

Bauman, Dale E., James W. Perfield II, Kevin J. Harvatine, and Lance H. BaumgardRegulation of Fat Synthesis by Conjugated Linoleic Acid: Lactation and the Ruminant Model. J. Nutr. February 2008. 138(2): 403-409.

Bell, A.W., 1995. *J. Anim. Sci.,* 73: 2804-2819.

Bell, A.W.; Bauman, D.E., 1997. *J. Mammary gland biology and Neoplasia*, 2: 265-278.

Bell, A.W; Burhans, W.S; Overton, T.R., 2000. *Proc. Nutr. Soc.*, 59: 119-136.

Ben-Ari, Y.; Cossart, R.; Kainte, 2000. *Trends.Neurosci.*, 23: 580-587.

Bennett CN, Knight CH and Wilde CJ.Regulation of mammary prolactin binding by a secreted milk protein. *J. Endocrinol* 1990; 127: S141.

Bezaire, V.; Hofmann, W.; Kramer, J.K.; Kozak, L.P.; Harper, M.E., 2001. *Am J Physiol Endocrinol, Metab.*, 281: E975-E982.

Block, S.S.; Butler, W.R.; Ehrhardt, R.A.; Bell, A.W.; Van Amburgh, M.E.; Boisclair, Y.R., 2001. *J. Endocrinol.*, 171: 339-348.

Block, S.S.; Rhoads, R.P.; Bauman, D.E.; Ehrhardt, R.A.; McGuire, M.A.; Crooker, B.A.; Griinari, J.M.; Mackle, T.R.; Weber, W.J.; Van Amburgh, M.E.; Boisclair, Y.R., 2003. *J. Dairy Sci.*, 86: 3508-3515.

Block, S.S.; Smith, J.M.; Ehrhardt, R.A.; Diaz, M.C.; Rhoads, R.P.; Van Amburgh, M.E.; Boisclair, Y. R., 2003. *J. Dairy Sci.*, 86: 3206-3214.

Boccia, M.L.; Goursaud, A.P.; Bachevalier, J.; Anderson, K.D.; Pedersen, C.A., 2007. 52(3): 344-51.

Bodoh, G.W.; Battista, W.J.; Schultze, L.H.; Johnston, R.P., 1976. *Journal of Dairy Science*, 50: 1119-1123.

Boisclair, Yves R. Role of leptin in regulating metabolism in highly productive ruminants CALS Impact Statement. http://vivo.cornell.edu/display/individual16530.

Book on Biology of lactation by GH Schmidt (1971), Publisher W H Freeman & Co., San Franscisco.

Book on Lactation Edited by B L Larson (1985), Publisher-Iowa Univ. Press, Iowa.

Bosch, O.J., 2012. *Horm. Behav.*, 61(3): 293-303. doi: 10.1016/j.yhbeh. 2011.11.002.

Bosch, O.J.; Meddle, S.L.; Beiderbeck, D.I.; Douglas, A.J.; Neumann, I.D.; 2005. *J. Neurosci.*, 25(29): 6807-15.

Bosch, O.J.; Neumann, I.D.; 2000. *Neurobiol*, 10: 784-9.

Boutinard, M.; Ben Chedly, M.H.; Delamaire, E.; Guinard- Flament, J., 2008. *J. Dairy Sci.*, 91: 988-998.

Bridges R.S.; Ronsheim, P.M., 1990. *Endocrinology*, 837-848.

Brogan, R.S.; Mitchell, S.E.; Trayhurn, P.; Smith, M.S., 1999. *Endocrinology*, 140: 2621-2628.

Broster, W.H., 1976. In *Principles of Cattle Production*, p. 271.

Bruckmaier, R.M.; 2003. *J. Dairy Res.*, 70, p. 123.

Bruckmaier, R.M.; Blum, J.W., 1998. *J. Dairy Sci.*, 81, pp 939.

Brumby, P.E.; Storry, J. E.; Bines, J.K.; Fulford, R.L., 1978. *Journal of Agriculture Science*, 91: 151-159.

Bruno, Stefanon; Monica, Colitti; Gianfranco, Gabai; Christopher, H.; Knightandcolin, J., 2002. *J.Dairy Research*, 69:1:37-52. • [PubMed] [Google Scholar] • szczensa-rundberg m [PubMed] [Google Scholar] • nielsen c [PubMed] [Google Scholar]

Brunton, P.J.; McKay.; Ochedalski, T.; et.al., 2009. *J.Neurosci.*, 29: 6449-6460.

Buijs, R.M., 1978. *Cell Tissues Res*, 192: 423-35.

Burke, C.R.; Williams, Y.J.; Hofmann, L.; Kay, J.K.; Phyn, C.V.C.; Meier, S., 2010. *J. Dairy Sci.*, 92: accepted.

Butler, S.T.; Marr, A.L.; Pelton, S.H.; Radcliff, R.P.; Lucy, M.C.; Butler, W.R., 2003. *J Endocrinol*, 176: 205-217.

Butler, W.R.; Smith, R.D., 1989. *J. Dairy Sci.*, 72: 767-783.

Byatt, J.C.; Sorbet, R.H.; Eppard, P.J.; Curran, T.L.; Curran, D.F.; Collier, R.J., 1992. *J. Dairy Sci.*, 75: 1216.

Capper, J.L.; Euridice, C.G.; Cady, R.A.; Dale E. Bauman., 2008. *Proc. Natl. Acad. Sci. USA*. 15; 105(28): 9668-9673. doi:10.1073/pnas. 0802446105.

Capuco, A.V.; Annen, E.; Fitzgerald, A.C.; Ellis, S.E.; Collier, R.J., 2006. In K. Sejrsen, T. Hvelplund, M.O. Nielsen, eds. Ruminant Physiology Wageningen Academic Publishers. The Netherlands, Pp. 363-387.

Carrasco G.A.; Van De Kar, L.D., 2003. *European Journal of Pharmacology*, 463(1-3): 259-284.

Carter, C.S.; Altemus, M., 1997. *Ann. N. Y. Acad. Sci.*, 807: 164-174.

Catherine Hebb and J.L. Linzell.1970. *Histochemical Journal*, 2(1970): 491-505.

Chaiyabutr, N., 1994. *Dairy cattle Newsletter*, 6(1): 3-4.

Chaiyabutr, N.; Komolvanich, S.; Preuksagorn, S.; Chanpongsang, S., 2000. *Asian-Austr. J. Anim. Sci.*, 13: 1359-1366.

Chaiyabutr, N.; Komolvanich, S.; Preuksagorn, S.; Chanpongsang, S., 2000. *Asian-Aus. J. Anim. Sci.*, 13(3): 334-347.

Champigny, O.; Ricquier, D., 1990. *J. Nutr.*, 120: 1730-1736.

Chang, T.H.; Kunasegaran, K.; Tarulli, G.A.; De Silva, D.; Voorhoeve, P.M.; Pietersen, A.M., 2014. *Breast Cancer Res.*, 7:16(1): R1.doi: 10.1186/bcr3593.

Chang, T.H.; Kunasegaran, K.; Tarulli, G.A.; De Silva, D.; Voorhoeve, P.M.; Pietersen, A.M.; 2014. Breast Cancer Res., 7:16(1): doi:10.1186/bcr3593.

Chilliard, Y.; Bonnet, M.; Delavaud, C.; Faulconnier, Y.; Leroux, C.; Djiane, J.; Bocquier, F., 2001. *Domest. Anim. Endocrinol.*, 21: 271-295.

Clark, D.A.; Phyn, C.V.C.; Tong, M.J.; Collis, S.J.; Dalley, D.E., 2006. *J. Dairy Sci.*, 89: 1854-1862.

Clevenger, C.V.; Chang, W.P.; Ngo, W.; Pasha, T.L.M.; Montone, K.T; Tomaszewski, J.E., 1995. *Am. J. Pathol.*, 46: 695-705.

Cole Barry, T.N., (1980). *N.Z. J. Agric. Res.*, 23: 427.

Cole, J.B.; Null, D.J., 2008. *J. Dairy sci.*, 92: 2248–2258; doi:10.3168/jds. 2008, 1825.

Collier, R.J.; Beede, D.K.; Thatcher, W.W.; Israel, L.A.; Wilcox, C.J., 1982a. *J. Dairy Sci.*, 65: 2213-2227.

Collier, R.J.; Dahl, G.E.; VanBaale, M.J., 2006. *J. Dairy Sci.*, 89: 1244-1253.

Collier, R.J.; Doelger, S.G.; Head, H.H.; Thatcher, W.W.; Wilcox, C.J., 1982b. *J. Anim. Sci.*, 54: 309-319.

Collier, R.J.; McNamara, J.P.; Wallace, C.R.; Dehoff; M.H.; 1984. *J. Anim. Sci.*, 59: 498-510.

Collier, R.J; Miller, M.A.; Hildebrandt, J.R.; Torkelson A.R.; *et al. J. Dairy Sci.*, 1991; 74: 2905-2911.

Connor, E.E..; Siferd, S.; Elsasser, T.H.; Clover, C.; Van Tassell, C.P.; Sonstegard, T.S.; Fernandes, V.; Capuco, A.V., 2008. *BMC genomics* doi: 10.1186/1471-2164-9-362.

Corah, L.R.; Lemenager, R.P.; Houghton, P.L.; Blasi, D.A., 1991. C-842. Kansas State University Agricultural Experiment Station and Cooperative Extension Service.

Cowie *et al.*, 1964, J. Endocrinol. 28:253 and 28:267.

Cowie, 1966. Anterior pituitary function in lactation. In The Pituitary Gland, Vol. 2, pp. 412-443, Eds. Harris and Donovan, Butterworths, London.

Cowie, 1966. *In The Pituitary Gland,* Vol. 2, pp. 412-443, Eds. Harris and Donovan, Butterworths, London.

Cowie, *et al.*, 1964. *J. Endocrinol.*, 28: 253-267.

Craven, N.; Williams, M.R., 1985. *Veterinary Immunol Immunopathology,* 10: 71.

Cristina Ovilo; Carmen Rodriguez Valdovinos. Http://www.eolss.net/Eolss-sampleallchapter.aspx.

Curley, K.O.; Neuendoff, D.A.; Lewis, A.W.; Rouquette, F.M.; Randel, R.D.; Welsh, T.H., 2010. *Physiology and Behavior,* 101(5): 699-704.

Curtis, S.E., 1983. Iowa State University Press, Ames, Iowa.

Dahl, G.E.; Buchanan, B.A.; Tucker, H.A.; 2000. *J. Dairy Sci.*, 83: 885-893.

Dahl, G.E.; Wallace, R.L.; Shanks, R.D.; Lueking, D., 2004. *J. Dairy Sci.,* 87: 882-885.

Dalley, D.E.; Clough, J.; Hofman, L.; Phyn, C.V.C.; Clark, D.A., 2008. *Proceedings of the New Zealand Society of Animal Production,* 68: 30-32.

Dang, A.K., Mahendra Singh and Anjuli Aggarwal (2002). Role of oxytocin in milk production and health of dairy animals- a review. *Indian Journal of Dairy Science,* 55(3): 191-198.

Dang, A.K., Singh, Mahendra and R.S. Ludri.1997. *Agric. Rev.,* 18: 201-211.

Dang, A.K.; Anand, S.K.; Singh, M., 2004. *Indian Dairyman,* 56(11): 27-32.

Derek LeRoith; Stefan Neuenschwander; Teresa L. Wood; Lothar Henninghausen., 1995. *Progress in Growth Factor Res.,* 6(2-4): 433-436.

Dewey, K.G., 1997. *Annu. Rev. Nutr.,* 17: 19-36.

Dijkman, J.T.; Lawrence, P.R., 1997. *J. Agric. Sci.,* 128: 95-103.

Djonov, V.; Andres, A. C.; Ziemiecki, A. 2001. *Microsc. Res. Tech.,* 52: 182-189.

Dohoo, I.R.; Meek, A.H., 1982. *Canadian Veterinary Journal,* 23: 119.

Drackley, J.K., 2001. *Proc. California Anim. Nutr. Conf. Fresno, CA. California Grain and Feed Assoc., Sacramento, CA.* Pp 113-134.

Eberhart, R.J.; Gilmore, H.C.; Hutchinson, L.J.; Spencer, S.B., 1979. *Proc National Mastitis Comp*, 32-40.

Elimam, A.; Lindgren, A.C.; Norgren, S.; Kamel, A.; Skwirut, C.; Bang, P.; Marcus, C., 1999. *Horm. Res.*, 52: 66-72.

Emery, R.S.; Liesman, J.S.; Herdt, T.H., 1992. *J. Nutr.*, 122: 832-837.

Eriksson, L.; Valtonen, M.; Laitinen, J.T.; Paananen, M.; Kaikkonen, M., 1998. *Acta Vet. Scand.*, 39(3): 301-310.

Escalada, J.; Cacicedo, L.; Ortego, J.; Melian, E.; Franco, F.S., 1997. *Endocrinol.*, 137: 631-637.

Exton, J.H., 1979. *In Hormones and Energy Metabolism,* p. 125.

Farooqi, I.S.; Matarese, G.; Lord, G.M.; Keogh, J.M.; Lawrence, E.; Agwu, C.; Sanna, V.; Jebb, S.A.; Perna, F.; Fontana, S.; Lechler, R.I.; DePaoli, A.M.; O'Rahilly S., 2002. *J. Clin. Invest.*, 110: 1093-1103.

Feldman, M.; Ruan, W.; Cunningham, B.C.; Wells, J.A.; Kleinberg, D.L., 1993. *Endocrinol.*, 133: 1602-1608.

Feuermann, Y.; Mabjeesh, S.J.; Shamay, A., 2004. *J.Dairy Sci.*, 87(9): 2941-2946.

Fields, K; Kulig, E.; Lloyd, R.V., 1993. *Lab. Invest*, 68: 354-360.

Finbar Mulligan; Luke O'Grady; Desmond Rice; Michael Doherty, 2006. *Irish Veterinary Journal*, 59(9): 506.

Flier, J.S., 1998. *J. Clin. Endocrinol. Metab.*, 83: 1407-1413.

Flint DJ and Knight CH Interactions of prolactin and growth hormone (GH) in the regulation of mammary gland function and epithelial cell survival. *Journal of Mammary Gland Biology and Neoplasia* 1997; 2: 41–48.

Forsyth, I.A.; Lee, P.D., 1993. *J. Dairy Res.*, 60(3): 307-17.

Fox, D.G.; Tylutki, T.P., 1998. *J. Dairy Sci.*, 81: 3085-3095.

Frandson, F.R., 1986. *Anatomy and physiology of farm animals.* Lea & Febiger, Philadelphia.

Garg, A.; Singh, M., 2008. *Indian Journal of Dairy Science,* 61(6): 465-467.

Garg, M.R.; Sherasia, P.L.; Bhandari, B.M.; Gulati, S.K.; Scott, T.W., 2002. *Indian Journal of Animal Nutrition,* 19: 191-198.

Garg, M.R.; Sherasia, P.L.; Bhandari, B.M.; Gulati, S.K.; Scott, T.W., 2003. *Animal Nutrition and Feed Technology,* 3: 151-157.

Geetha, E.; Chakravarty, A.K.; Vinaya, K., 2006. *Asian-aust. J. Anim. Sci.,* 19(12): 1696-1701.

Gengler, N., 1996. *Interbull Bull.,* 12: 87–96.

Gertler, A.; Ashkenazi, A.; Madar, Z., 1984. *Molecular and Cellular Endocrinol.,* 34: 51-57.

Glimm D.R., Baraces V.E.& Kennelly, J.E.1992. J. Dairy Sci., 75: 2687–2708.

Glimm, D.R.; Baracos, V.E.; Kennelly J.J., 1988. *J. Dairy Sci.,* 71: 2923-2935.

Glimm, D.R.; Baracos, V.E.; Kennelly, J.J., 1990. *J. Endocrinol.,* 126: R5.

Gnanasekar, R., Mahendra Singh, Ashwani Kumar Roy Ajithakumar, H.M. and Sunita Thakur. 2016.

Goff, J.P., 2003. *Cattle Practice,* 11(2): 51-63.

Groenewegen, P.P.; McBride, B.W.; Burton, J.H.; Elsasser, T.H, 1990. *J.Nutr.,* 120: 514-520.

Grum, D.E.; Drackley, J.K.; Clark, J.H., 2002. *J. Dairy Sci.,* 85: 3026-3034.

Grum, D.E.; Drackley, J.K.; Younker, R.S.; LaCount, D.W.; Veenhuizen, J.J., 1996. *J. Dairy Sci.,* 79: 1850-1864.

Guinard-Flament, J.; Delamaire, E.; Lemonsquet, S.; Boutinard, M.; David, Y., 2006. *Reproduction, nutrition and development,* 46: 589-598.

Guinard-Flament, J.; Delamaire, E.P.; Lamberton, P.; Peyraud. J.L., 2007. *J. Dairy Sci.,* 90: 5062-5072.

Hale, S.A.; Capuco, A.V.; Erdman, R.A., 2003. *J. Dairy Sci.,* 86: 2061-2071.

Hallen, S.C.; Waller, P.; Emanuelson, U., 2008. *Veterinary Journal,* 175(1): 108-117.

Hammond, A.C.; Olson, T.A. chase, C.C.; *et al.,* 1996. *J. Ani. Sci.,* 74(2): 295-303.

Hansson, H.; Szczensa-Rundberg, M.; Nielsen, C., 2010. doi: 10.1017/S1751731110002247 Published online by Cambridge University Press.

Haque, Nilufar, Mahendra Singh and S.A. Hossain, 2015. *International J. Dairy Sci.,* 10: 95-106.

Haque, Nilufar, Mahendra Singh, Sheikh Asraf Hossain. 2016. *Intn. J. Biometrologty*, 60: 1819–1828.

Hardin, R., 1990. C-817. University of Georgia College of Agricultural and Environmental Sciences, Cooperative Extension Service.

Harvatine KJ, Boisclair YR, Bauman DE. Recent advances in the regulation of milk fat synthesis. Animal. 2009 Jan;3(1):40-54. doi: 10.1017/S1751731108003133.

Heaton, M.P.; Grosse, W.M.; Kappes, S.M.; Keele, J.W.; Chitko-McKown, C.G.; 2001. *Mamm. Genome.*, 12: 32-37.

Heinford, B.W.; Shum–Siu, A.; Leonberger, M.; Hendler, F.J., 1993. *Nucleic Acids Res.*, 21: 3159-3166.

Henry, B.A.; Goding, J.W.; Alexander, W.S.; Tilbrook, A.J.; Canny, B.J.; Dunshea, F.; Rao, A.; Mansell, A.; Clarke, J., 1999. *Endocrinol.*, 140: 1175-1182.

Henry, J.P., 1993. *NIPS* 8: 69-73.

Hernandez. Evaluation of serotonin as feed back inhibition of lactation. *Jouranal of Dairy Science* 2008; (44): 1834-1846.

Heuwieser, W.; Tenhagen, B.A.; Tischer, M.; Luhr, J.; Blum H., 2000. *Vet. Rec.* 146: 338-341.

Hogan, J.S.; Smith, L.L. 1987. *Comp Continuing Educ Pract Vet,* 9: 341.

Holcomb, C.S.; Van Horn, H.H.; Head, H.H.; Hall, M.B.; Wilcox, C.J., 2001. *J. Dairy Sci.,* 84: 2051-2058.

Holmes, C.W.; Kamote, H.; Mackenzie, D.D.; Morel, P.C.H., 1996. *Australian Journal of Dairy Technology,* 51: 8-11.

Holtenius, K.; Agenas, S.; Delavaud, C.; Chilliard, Y., 2003. *J. Dairy Sci.,* 86: 883-891.

Hooley, R.D., J.J. Campbell, and J.K. Findlay. 1978. J. Endocrinol. 79: 301-310.

http://ansci.illinois.edu/static/ansc438/Milkcompsynth/milksynth_fatsources.html

Indian J. Anim. Nutr. 33 (4): 399-403.

Ingvartsen, K.L.; Boisclair, Y.R., 2001. *Domest. Anim. Endocrinol.,* 21: 215-250.

Isaksson, O.G., Eden, S.and Jansson, J.O. 1985. *Annual Rev. Physiol.,* 47: 483–499.

Itoh, F.; Obara, Y.; Fuse, H.; Osaka, I.; Hodate, K., 1997. *Anim.Sci. Technol.,* (Jpn.) 68: 727-734.

Itoh, F.; Obara, Y.; Rose, M.T.; Fuse, H.; Hashimoto, H., 1998. *J. Anim.Sci.,* 76: 2182-2189.

Iwasaka, T.; Shinobu, U.; Kochi K.; Haruko K.; Yoshiyuki, R.O., ·2000. *J. Histochem. Cytochem.* 48: 389-396.

Jaymelynn, K. Farney; Laman, K. Mamedova; Johann, F. Coetzee; Butch KuKanich, Lorraine M. Sordillo; Sara, K. Stoakes; Ernest, Minton J.; Larry, C. Hollis; Barry, J. Bradford, 2013. *Am. J. Physiol. Regul. Integr. Comp. Physiol.,* 15; 305(2): R110–R117.

Jenkins, T.C.; Palmquist, D.L., 1984. *J. Dairy Sci.,* 67: 978-986.

Jeremy, T. Smith; Peter, J. Mark; Brendan, J. Waddell, 2005. *J. Endocrinol.,* 184: 535-541.

Jindal, S.K.; Mahendra Singh; Ludri, R.S., 1988. *Indian Dairyman,* 40(2): 83-84.

Jingar, S.C.; Mehla, R.K.; Singh, M.; Kumar, A.; Kantwa, S.C.; *et.al.,* 2014. *Indian Journal of Animal Research,* 48(2): 194-197.

Jingar, S.C.; Mehla, R.K.; Singh, M.; Singh, P.K., 2014. *Journal of Bio Innovation,* 3(3): 117-123.

Johnson, L.R.; Farb, C.; Morrison, J.H.; McEwen, B.S.; LeDoux, J.E., 2005. *Neuroscience,* 136(1): 289-299.

Johnsson, I. D., 1988. In: Nutrition and Lactation in the Dairy Cow, pp. 171-192 [P. C. Garnsworthy, editor]. London: Butterworth.

Jonathan, N.B.; Mershon, J.L.; Allen, D.L; Steinmetz, R.W., 1996. Endocrine Rev., 17: 639-669.

Joydip Mukherjee, Mandira Chaudhury and Kalyan De. 2011.Feed Back Inhibition of Lactation: An Autocrine Regulator of Milk Secretion., 6(2): Article 86.

Joydip Mukherjee; Mandira Chaudhury; Kalyan De, 2011. 6(2): Article 86.

Jyotsna Prasad; Mahendra Singh., 2010. *Agric. Biol. J.N. Am.,* 1(6): 1325-1327.

Jyotsna, Prasad; Mahendra, Singh, 2001. *Asian Austrlasian J. Animal Scenes,* 41(5): 684-692.

Jyotsna; Mahendra Singh, 2010. *Agric. Biol. J. N. Am.,* 1(6): 1325-1327.

Kadzere, C.T.; Murphy, M.R.; Silanikove, N.; Maltz, E., 2002. *Livestock Production Science,* 77: 59-91.

Kathleen, J. Motil; Mary, T. Corinne; Montandon, M.; David, H; Thomas, W; Boaoetton, Klein, P.D.; Caoetbertogarza. 2009. *J. Nutrition. Org.*

Kaushal, S. 2013. Persistency of milk yield in Sahiwal Cattle. Thesis submitted to the National Dairy Research Institute, Karnal (Deemed University).

Kay, J.K.; Phyn, C.V.C.; Williams, Y.J.; Roche, J.R.; Burke, C.R.; Meier, S., 2009. *Proceedings of the New Zealand Society of Animal Production,* 69: 24-26.

Kazmer, G.W.; Barnes, M.A.; Akers, R.M.; Whittier, W.D., 1986. *J. Endocrinol.,* 109: 175.

Keeanan, T.W.; Morre, J.T.; Huang, C.M., 1974. Membranes of the mammary gland. In: *Lactation.* Vol. II. Eds. B.L. Larson & V.R. Smith. Academic Press, New York.

Kendrick, K.; Keverne, E.; 1992. *Ann NY Acad Sci.,* 652: 102-121.

Keys, J.E. and Djiane, J. 1988. J. Receptor Res., 8: 731–750.

Khan-dawood, F.S.; Ayromlooi, J.; Tobias, M., 1983. *Am. J. Obstet. Gynecol.,* 147(5): 584-588.

Kinsley, C.H.; Lambert, K.G., 2008. *J Neuroendocrinol,* 20: 515-25.

Kitchen, B.J., 1981. *Journal of Dairy Research,* 48: 167-188.

Klachko, D.H.; Anderson R.R.; Heimberg, M., New York: Plenum Press.

Kleinberg, D.L., Ruan, W., Catanese, V., Newman, C.B.and Feldman, M.1990. *Endocrinol.,* 126: 3274–3276.

Kleppe, B.B.; Aiello, R.J.; Grummer, R.R.; Armentano, L.E., 1988. *J. Dairy Sci.,* 71: 1813-1822.

Knaggs, G.S., 1967. *Journal of Endocrinology,* 37: 229-230.

Knight, C.H., 2000. *Livestock Prod. Sci.,* 66: 169-176.

Knight, C.H.; Calvert, D.T.; Flint, D.J., 1986. *J. Endocr.,* 110: 263-270.

Knight, C.H.; Docherty, A.H.; Peaker, M., 1984. *J. Dairy Res.,* 51: 29-36.

Knight, C.H.; Hirst, D.; Dewhurst, R.J., 1994. *J. Dairy Res.,* 61, p.167.

Knight, C.H.; Peaker, M., 1984. *Q. J. Exp. Physiol.,* 69: 331-338.

Knight, C.H.; Peaker, M.; 1982. *J. Reprod. Fert.,* 65: 521-536.

Knight, C.H.; Peaker, M.; Colin, J.W., 1998. *Reviews of Reprod.*, 3: 104-112.

Knight, C.H.; Wilde, C. J., 1987. *J. Dairy Sci.*, 70(9): 1991-2000.

Knight, C.H.; Wilde, C.J., 1988. *J. Dairy Res.*, 55: 487-493

Knight, C.H.; Wilde, C.J., 1993. *Liv. Prod. Sci.*, 35: 3-19.

Knight, K.C. and M. Peaker. 1984. Quarterly J. Expt. Physiol. 69: 331.

Knowlton, K.F.; Dawson, T.E.; Glenn, B.P.; Huntington, G.B.; Erdman, R.A., 1998. *J. Dairy Sci.*, 81: 3248-3258.

Kossaibati, M.A.; Esslemont, R.J., 1997. *Vet. J.*, 154: 41-51.

Kumud, N.K.; Prakash, B.S., 2001. *Buffalo J.* 3, p. 34.

Kurtz, A.; Bristol, L.A.; Toth, B.E.; Lazar–Wesley, E.; Takacs, L.; Kacsoh, B., 1993. *Biol. Reprod.*, 48: 1095-1103.

Lacy-Hulbert, S.J.; Dalley, D.E.; Clark, D.A., 2005. *Proceedings of the New Zealand Society of Animal Production,* 65: 137-142.

Laura, K.; Ramos, J.G.; Hugo, H.O.; Gregorio, S.M; Leonardo, E.B.; Enrique, H.L.; Monica, M. de Toro., 2001. *Endocrinol.* 5: 263-269.

Lay, D.C.; Friend, T.H.; Randel, R.D.; Bowers, C.L.; Grissom, K.K.; Jenkins, O.C., 1992. *J Ani Sci.*, 70(2): 330-336.

Le Blanc, S.J.; Leslie, K.E.; Duffield, T.F., 2005. *J. Dairy Sci.*, 88: 159-170.

Lee, C.S., Wooding, F.B.P.; Kemp, P., 1980. *Journal of Dairy Research,* 47: 39.

Lee, J.K.; Won, J.S.; Singh, A.K.; Singh, I., 2008. *Neurosci Lett,* 440: 260-4.

Lefcourt, M.; Akers, R.M., 1983. *J. Dairy Sci.*, 66, p. 2251.

Lewis, G.S., 1997. *J. Dairy Sci.*, 80: 984-994.

Lincoln, D.T., Sinowatz, F., El-Hifnawi, E., Hughes, R.L.and Waters, M. 1995. Anatomia, Histologia, Embryologia 24: 107–115.

Lincoln, G.A.; Clarke, I.J., 1995. *J. Neuroendocrinol.*, 7: 637-643.

Lkhider, M.; Delpal, S.; Bousquet, M.O., 1996. *Endocrinol.*, 137: 4969-4979.

Loffreda, S.; Yang, S.Q.; Lin, H.Z.; Karp, C.L.; Brengman, M.L.; Wang, D.J.; Klein, A.S.; Bulkley, G.B.; Bao, C.; Noble, P.W.; Lane, M.D.; Diehl. A.M., 1998. *The FASEB Journal,* 12: 57-65.

Lomax, M.A.; Baird, G.D.; Mallinson, C.B.; Symonds, H.W., 1979. *Biochem. J.*, 180: 281-289.

Lowenberg, M.; Stahn, C.; Hommes, D.W.; Buttgereit, F.; 2008. *Steroids,* 73(9-10): 1025-1029.

Lucy, M.C., 2000. *J. Dairy Sci.,* 83: 1635-1647.

Ludri, R.S. and Mahendra Singh. 1987. Milk production, dry matter and water consumption of crossbred cows milked with and without oxytocin. Indian Journal of Animal Sciences. 57: 778-780.

Ludri, R.S.; Mahendra Singh 1989. *International J. Ani. Sci.,* 4: 52-55.

Ludri, R.S.; Mahendra Singh, 1987. *Indian J. Ani. Sci.,* 57: 1310-1313.

Ludri, R.S.; Mahendra Singh., 1989. *Asian Livestock,* 7: 78-80.

Ludri, R.S.; Upadhyay, R.C.; Mahendra Singh; Guneratne, J.R.; Basson, R.P., 1989. *J. Dairy Sci.,* 72: 2283-2287.

MacRae, J.C.; Lobley, G.E., 1982. *Livestock Production Science,* 9: 447-456.

Mahendra Singh and A.K. Dang. 2002. Does oxytocin affect milk production and reproduction of dairy animals. *Indian Dairyman,* 54(4): 65-69.

Mahendra Singh and Anjuli Aggarwal. 2001. Effect of oxytocin administration on certain minerals in the milk of buffaloes. *Asian-Australasian J. Animal Sciences,* (Korea), 14(11): 1523-1526.

Mahendra Singh and Prakash, B. S. 2013. *Indian J. Anim. Sci.,* 83(63): 615-617.

Mahendra Singh, A.K. Roy and Shikha Sharma, 2015. *Asian J. Anim. & Vety. Adv.* 10: 476-488.

Mahendra Singh, Anjali Aggarwal and S. Mallick. 2016. *Indian J. Anim. Res.,* 50 (1) 2016: 123-128.

Mahendra Singh.2011. Oxytocin: The cuddle Hormone-A Review. *Agric. Rev.,* 32(4): 294-303.

Mahendra Singh; A.K. Dang; Anjuli Aggarwal., 2001. *Indian J.Anim. Prod. & Managt.,* 17: 49-53.

Mahendra Singh; A.K. Dang; Anjuli Aggarwal., 2002. *Indian J. Dairy Sci.,* 55(6): 342-345.

Mahendra Singh; Ludri, R.S., 1994. *Buffalo J.,* 10: 81-84.

Mahendra Singh; Ludri, R.S., 1999. *Asian-Australasian J. Anim.Sci.,* 12: 585-589.

Mahendra Singh; R.S. Ludri., 1999. *Small Rumi. Res.,* 31: 141-147.

Mahendra Singh; R.S. Ludri., 2000. *Small Rumi. Res.*, 35: 255-262.

Mahendra Singh; R.S. Ludri., 2002. *Asian Australasian J. Anim. Sci.*, 15(7): 963-967.

Mahendra, Singh; Ludri, R.S., 2001. *Asian-Australasian J. Animal Sciences,* 14 (12): 1775-1780.

Mahendra, Singh; Ludri, R.S., 2001. *Asian-Australasian Journal of Animal Sciences,* 41(2): 189-192.

Mahmoud, K.G.M.; M.F., 2012. *Iranian Journal of Applied Animal Science,* 2(3): 203-222.

Marcek, J.M.; Swanson, L.V., 1984. *J. Dairy Sci.,* 67: 2380-2388.

Marcus, E.K.; Dale, E.S., 1994. *Journal of Dairy Science,* 77: 619-627.

Margaret C. Neville; Thomas B. McFadden; Isabel Forsyth, 2002. *J. Mammary Gland Biology and Neoplasia,* 7(1): 49-66.

Margaret, C. Neville; Daniel, M.; Jenifer, M.; Russel, R.C., 2004. *J. Mammary Gland Biol. and Neoplasia,* 3(2): 109-116.

Mario Baratta. Role of Leptin in the Mammary Gland Development, Lactation and in Neonatal Physiology pp. 89-106, *Veterinary Physiology, University of Turin, Italy.*

Martin, T. Sorensen; Hacker R.R., 1979. *J. Anim. Sci.,* 49: 1270-1275.

Matarese, G.; Moschos, S; Christos S. Mantzoros, 2005. J. Immunology, 174: 3137-3142.

McEwan, A.D.; Fisher, E.W.; Selman, I.E., 1970. *Clinical Chemistry Acta,* 17: 155.

McEwen, B.S.; The brain as a target of endocrine hormones. In Neuroendocrinology. Krieger and Hughs, Eds.: 33-42. Sinauer Association, Inc., Massachusetts, 1980.

McGuire, M.A.; Beede, D.E.; Delorenzo, M.A.; Wilcox, C.J.; Huntington, G.B.; Reynolds,C.K.; Collier, R.J., 1989. *J. Anim. Sci.,* 67: 1050-1060.

McGuire, M.A.; Griinari, J.M.; Dwyer, D.A.; Bauman, D.E., 1995. *J. Dairy Sci.,* 78: 816-824.

McNamara, S.; Murphy, J.J.; O'Mara, F.P.; Rath, M.; Mee, J.F., 2008. *Liv. Sci.,* 117: 70-78.

Megan, Galbally; Andrew, J. Lewis; Marinus, van Ijzendoorn; Michael, Permezel, 2012. http://www.marinusvanijzendoorn.nl/wp.

Mershon, J.; Sall, W.; Mitchner, N.; Jonathan, N.B., 1995. *Endocrinol.,* 136: 2619-2623.

Michael, P. Heaton; Gregory, P. Harhay; Gary, L. Bennett; Roger, T. Stone; Michael Grosse,W.; Eduardo, Casas; John, W. Keele; Timothy, P.L. Smith; Carol, G. Chitko-McKown; William, W. Laegreid, 2002. *Mamm. Genome.,* 13: 272-281.

Mizuno, H.; Sensui, N., 1970. *Endocrinol. Japan* 17: 417.

Momongan, V.G.; Schmidt, G.H., 1970. *J. Dairy Sci.,* 53: 747-751.

Mor Kobayashi, Y.; Boyd, C.K.; McCormack, B.L.; Lucy, M.C., 2002. *J. Dairy Sci.,* 85: 748-754.

Moran, C.; Quirke, J.F.; Roche, J.F., 1989. *Anim. Reprod. Sci.,* 18: 167-162.

Muriel, Bonnet; Carole, Delavaud; Karine, Laud; Isabelle, Gourdou; Christine, Leroux; Jean, Djiane; Yves, Chilliard; 2002. *Reprod. Nutr. Dev.,* 42: 399-413 (DOI: 10.1051/rnd:2002034).

Mustafa, M.Y.; Saleem, K.; Munir, R.; Butt, T.M., 2008. *Livestock Research for Rural Development,* 20(12):

Nardone, A.; Lacetera, N.; Bernabucci, U.; Ronchi, B., 1997. *J. Dairy Sci.,* 80: 838-844.

National Research Council, 1981. *National Academy Press, Washington, DC,* Pages 75-84.

Neeru and Singh, Mahendra. 1995. *Indian J.Dairy Sci.,* 48: 216-222.

Neeru and Singh, Mahendra. 1997. *Indian Vet. J.,* 74:652-654.

Neeru and Singh, Mahendra. 1997. *Indian J.Prod. Mgmt.,* 13: 39-42.

Newbould, F.H.S., 1978. *Journal of Food production,* 41: 96-99.

Newton, M.; Newton, N.R., 1948. *J.Pediatr.,* 33: 698-704.

Norgaard, J.; Sorensen, A.; Sorensen, M.T.; Andersen, J.B.; Sejrsen, K., 2005. *J. Dairy Sci.,* 88: 975-982.

Numan, M.; Fleming, A.S; Levy, F., 2006. Maternal Behaviour. In: Neill JD, Ed. Knobil and Neill's physiology of reproduction. 3rd ed. Amsterdam, Boston: Elsevier, 2006.

O'callaghan, D.; Karsch, F.J.; Boland, M.P.; Roche, J.F., 1991. *Biol. Reprod.,* 44: 23-28.

Olins, G.M.; Bremel, R.D., 1984. *Endocrinol.,* 114: 1617-1626.

Oliphint, R.A.; Evaluation of the inter-relationships of temperament, stress responsiveness and immune function in beef calves, M.S. thesis, Texas A & M university , college station, 2006.

Ostrowska, Z.; Kos-Kudla, B.; Swietochowska, E.; Marek, B.; Kajdaniuk, D.; Ciesielskakopacz, N., 2001. *Neuroendocrinol. Lett.*, 22: 255-262.

Parodi P.W., 2005. *J. AM. COLL. Nutr.*, 24(6 Suppl): 556S-68S. http:// www.jacn.org/content/24/ suppl_6/ 556S.long.

Patial, M.P.; Nagvekar, A.S.; Ingole, S.D.; Bharucha, S.; Palve, V.T., 2015. *Veterinary World*, 8(3): 363-366.

Patton, J.; Kenny, D.A.; Mee, J.F.; O'Mara, F.P.; Wathes, D.C.; Cook, M.; Murphy, J.J., 2006. *J. Dairy Sci.*, 89: 1478-1487.

Paul, D.; Walden, W.R.; Mark, F.; David, L.K., 1998. *Endocrinol.*, 139(2): 659-662.

Pedraza, N.; Solanes, G.; Iglesias, R.; Vazquez, M.; Giralt, M.; Villarroya, F., 2001. *Biochem. J.*, 355: 105–111.

Pekka, Uimari; Anu, Sironen; Marja-Liisa, Sevon-Aimonen, 2011. *Genetics Selection Evolution*, 43: 42.

Perry, N.A.; Doon, R.J., 1950. *Journal of Dairy Science*, 33: 176.

Person, K.; Sandgren, C.H.; Rodriguez, M., 1992. *American Journal of Veterinary Research*, 53: 2235.

Peters, R.R.; Chapin, L.T.; Emery, R.S.; Tucker, H.A., 1981. *J. Dairy Sci.*, 64: 1671-1678.

Peters, R.R.; Chapin, L.T.; Leining, K.B.; Tucker, H.A., 1978. *Science*, 199: 911-912.

Petitclerc *et al.*, 1985. *J. Dairy Sci.*, 68: 86.

Pfeilsticker, H.U.; Bruckmaier, R.M.; Blum, J.W., 1995. *J. Dairy Res.*, 62, p. 559.

Phyn, C.V.C.; kay, J.K.; Rius, A.G.; Davis, S.R.; Stelwagen, K.; Hillerton, J.E.; Roche, J.R., 2010. *Proceedings of the 4th Australasian Dairy Sci. Sympos.*, 156-164.

Pinillia, L.; Tena-sempere, M.; Aguilar, R.; Aguilar, E., 1998. *Eur J. Endocrinol.*, 138: 460-466.

Pitt, G.R.; Batt, A.R.; Haigh, R.M.; Penson, A.M.; Robson, P.A.; Rooker, D.P.; Tartar, A.L.; Trim, J.E.; Yea, C.M.; Roe, M.B., 2004. *Bioorganic & Medicinal Chemistry Letters*, 14: 4585-4589.

Plotsky, P.M.; 1991. *Journal of Neuroendocrinology,* 3(1): 1-9.

Prakash, B.S.; Metten, M.; Schams, D.; Wuttke, W.; 1998. *Anim. Reprod. Sci.,* 51, p. 185.

Prasad, J.; Singh, M., 2001. *Asian Austrlasian Journal of Animal Sciences,* 41(5): 684-692.

Prosser, C.G.; Fleet, I.R.; Davis, A.J.; Heap, R.B., 1991. *J. Endocrinol.,* 131: 459-466.

Prosser, C.G.; Royle, C.; Fleet, I.R.; Mepham, T.B., 1991. *J. Endocrinol.,* 128: 457-463.

Provost, F.L.; Leroux, C.; Martin, P.; Gaye, P.; Djiane, J., 1994. *Neuroendocrinol,* 60: 305-313.

Purup, S.; Sejrsen, K.; Foldager, J.; Akers, R.M., 1993. *J. Endocrinol.,* 139: 19-26.

Purup, S.; Sejrsen. K.; Akers, R.M., 1993. *Livestock Prod. Sci.,* 35: 182-183.

Quinn, T., 1980. Dairy farm management. Van Nostrand Reinhold, New York.

Ragnauth, A.K.; Devidze, N.; Moy, V.; et.al., 2005. *Brain.Behav.,* 4: 229-239.

Rahman, Z.; Resnick, L.; Rosenzweig-lipson, S.J.; Ring, R.H.; *US patent application* 2007/0117794, published 2007-05-24, assigned to WYETH Corp.

Rayner, V.C.; Robinson, I.C.; Russell, J.A., 1995. *Journal Physiol.,* 396: 319-347.

Reiter, R.J., 1991. *Trends. Endocrin. Met.,* 2: 13-29.

Reksen, O.; Tverdal, A.; Landsverk, K.; Kommisrud, E.; Boe, K.E.; Ropstad, E., 1999. *J. Dairy Sci.,* 82: 810-816.

Remond, B.; Aubailly, S.; Chilliard, Y.; Dupont, D.; Pomies, D.; Petit, M., 2002. *Animal Research,* 51: 101-117.

Remond, B.; Pomies, D.; Dupont, D.; Chilliard, Y., 2004: *Animal Research,* 53: 201-212.

Remond. B.; Pomies, D., 2005. *Animal Research,* 54: 427-442.

Report (1999) on the Food and Drug Administration's: Review of the Safety of Recombinant Bovine Somatotropin"http://www.fda.gov/AnimalVeterinary/SafetyHealth/ProductSafetyInformation/ucm130321.htm.

Reynolds, C.K., 2005. *Proceedings of Florida Ruminant Nutrition Symposium* p. 143-154.

Rhen T.; Cidlowski, J.A.; 2005. *New England Journal of Medicine,* 353(16): 1711-1658.

Rhoads, R.P.; *et al.,* 2007. *J. Endocrinol.,* 195: 49-58.

Rison, C.D.; Daniel, J.A.; Holmberg, B.J.; Djiane, J.; Raver, N.; Gertler, A.; Keisler, D.H., 2001. *J. Endocrinol.,* 168: 317-324.

Rius, A.G.; Kay, J.K.; Phyn, C.V.C.; Morgan, S.R.; Roche, J.R., 2010. *J. Dairy Sci.,* 93 (Supplement 1): accepted abstract.

Robinson, J.J., 1990. *Nutr. Res. Rev.,* 3: 253-276.

Roche, J.R., 2007. *Liv. Sci.,* 110: 12-24.

Röpke R, Sauerwein H, Stoel B, Hagen-Mann K, von Ahnen S & Meyer HHD. J. Reprod. & Develop., 40: 227–234.

Rulofson, F.C.; Brown, D.E.; Bjur, R.A., 1998. *J. Ani Sci,* 66(5): 1223-1229.

Saha, A.; Mahendra Singh., 1998. *Asian-Australasian J. Anim.Sci.,* 11(4): 368-374.

Sanno, N.; Jin, L.; Qian, X.; Osamura, R.Y.; Scheithauer, B.W.; Kovacs, K.; Lloyd, R.V., 1997. *J. Clinical Endocrinol. & Metab.,* 82: 1974-1982.

Sano, H.; Lee, S.R.; Yamazaki, F.; Orlandi, M.; Sasaki, Y.; Tsuda, T., 1988. *Jpn. J. Zootech. Sci.,* 59: 1019-1026.

Sapino, A.; Macri, L.; Tonda, L.; Bussolati, G., 1993. *Endocrinol.,* 133: 838-842.

Sapolsky, R.M.; Romero, L.M.; Munck, A.U.; 2000. *Endocrine Reviews,* 21(1): 55-89.

Sartin, J. L.; Cummins, K.A.; Kemppainen, R.J.; Marple, D.N.; Rahe, C.H.; Williams, J.C., 1985. *Am. J. Physiol.,* 248: E108-E114.

Sastry, G.A., 1978. Clinical veterinary pathology, 2nd edition (CBS Publisher and Distributors. Delhi).

Schams, D., *Acta Endocrinol,* (Copenh.). 103, p. 180.

Schams, D., Acta Endocrinol. (Copenh.) 103 (1983), p. 180. Full Text via CrossRef | View Record in Scopus | Cited By in Scopus (55).

Schillo, K.K.; Hall, J.B.; Hileman, S.M., 1992. *J. Anim. Sci.,* 70: 3994-4005.

Schlamberger, G.; Wiedemann, S.; Vitrro, E.; Meyer, H.H.D.; Kaske, M., 2010. *J. Dairy Sci.,* 93: 2471-2485.

Schreiner, D.A.; Ruegg, P.L., 2003. *J. Dairy Sci.*, 86: 3460-3465. Shultz, T.A.; Morrison, S.R., 1987. *Calif. Agric.*, 41: 12-13.

Schultz, L.H., 1977. *Journal of Animal* and *Veterinary Medicine*, 170: 1244-1246.

Sejrsen, K., 1978. *Acta Agri. Scandinavica*, 28: 4146.

Sejrsen, K.; Foldager, J.; Sorensen, M.T.; Akers, R.M.; Bauman, D.E., 1986. *J. Dairy Sci.*, 69: 1528-1538.

Sejrsen, K.; Huber, J.T.; Tucker, H.A., 1983. *J. Diary Sci.*, 66: 845-855.

Sejrsen, K.; Huber, J.T.; Tucker, H.A.; Akers, R.M., 1982. *J. Dairy Sci.*, 65: 783-800.

Shailja; Mahendra Singh, 2002. *Asian-Australasian J. Animal Sciences*, 15(10): 1517-1522.

Shamay, A.; Cohen, N.; Niwa, M.; Gertler, A., 1988. *Endocrinol.*, 123: 804-809.

Shani, J.; Knaggs, G.S.; Tindal, J.S., 1971. *J. Endocrinol.*, 50: 543.

Sharma, N., 2007. Review, *Asian Journal of Animal* and *Veterinary Advances*, 2(2): 50-62.

Sharma, N.; Singh, N.K.; Bhadwal, M.S., 2011. *Asian Australasian Journal of Animal Science*, 24(3): 429-438.

Sharma, Shika , Mahendra Singh, A.K. Roy and S. Thakur. 2016. *Vet. World*, 9(3): 256-259.

Sharma, Shika and Mahendra Singh. 2016. *Indian J. Anim. Research*, DOI:10.18805/ijar.9637.

Shipe, W.F.; Senyk, G.F.; Fountain, K.B., 1980. *Journal of Dairy Science*, 65: 193-198.

Silva, I.D.; Silva, K.F.S., 1994. *Buffalo Journal*, 2: 133-137.

Singh, M.; Dang, A.K.; Prasad, P., 2001. *Indian Dairyman*, 53(6): 45-48.

Singh, M.; Ludri, R.S., 1999. Somatic cell counts in milk of buffaloes, (Proceedings National Seminar on sustainable developments of buffaloes for milk, meat and draft, held at NDRI) 17.

Singh, M.; Ludri, R.S., 2001. *Asian Australasian Journal of Animal Sciences*, 41(2): 189-192.

Singh, Mahendra and Kumar, P. 1994. *Indian Vet. J.* 71: 405.

Singh, Mahendra, Ludri, R.S. and Nair, S. 1994. *Indian J.Dairy Sci.*, 47: 708-711.

Singh, Mahendra, Ludri, R.S. and Nair, S. 1995. *Indian J. Prod. Mgmt.* 11: 54-57.

Singh, Mahendra, Nair, S., Ludri, R.S. and Seth, R. 1994. *Indian Vet. J.* 71: 524-525.

Singh, Mahendra, R.P. Singh and Omvir Singh.2000. *Indian Vet. J.*, 77: 237-239.

Singh, Mahendra, Verma, G.S. and Ludri, R.S. 1997. *Indian Vet. J.*, 74: 979-980.

Singh, Mahendra; Dang, A.K., 2006. *Livestock International*, 7: 11-14.

Singh, Mahendra; Dey, R.A.; Sharma, D.K., 2007. *Indian Dairyman*, 60: 40-44.

Singh, Mahendra; Ludri, R.S., 1994. *Buffalo J.*, 10: 81-84.

Singh, Mahendra; Ludri, R.S., 1999. *Small Rum. Res.*, 31: 141-147.

Singh, Mahendra; Sharma, D.K.; Dutta S.; Ghosh, A., 2008. *Indian J. Dairy Sci.*, 61(4): 295-297.

Singh, Mahendra; Tyagi, A.K.; Mehla, R.K.; Charan, S., 2003. *Indian J. Ani. Sci.*, 73(6): 117.

Singhal, O.P.; Des Raj, 1989. *Indian Dairyman*, 41: 43-47.

Sivitz, W.I.; Fink, B.D.; Donohoue, P.A.; 1999. *Endocrinology*, 140: 1511-1519.

Sivitz, W.I.; Fink, B.D.; Morgan, D.A.; Fox, J.M.; Donohoue, P.A.; Haynes, W.G., 1999. *Am. J. Physiol. Endocrinol. Metab.*, 277: E668-E677.

Skaar, T.C.; Grummer, R.R.; Dentine, M.R.; Stauffacher, R.H., 1989. *J. Dairy Sci.*, 72: 2028-2038.

Skrundz, M.; Bolten, M.; Nast, I.; Hellhammer, D.H., 2011. *Neuro-psychopharmacology*, 36: 1886-1893.

Smith, K.L.; Waldron, M.R.; Overton, T.R.; Drackley, J.K.; Socha, M.T., 2002. *J. Dairy Sci.*, 85(Suppl. 1): 23.

Smith, M.S.; Grove, K.L., 2002. *Front Neuroendocrinol.*, 23: 225-256.

Smith, V.G.; Beck, T.W.; Convey, E.M., 1974. *Neuro endocrinology*, 15: 172-181.

Smith, V.G.; Beck, T.W.; Convey, E.M.; Tucker H.A., 1974. *Neuroendocrinology*, 15(3-4): 172-181.

Smoak K. A.; Cidlowski, J.A. 2008. *NeuroImmune Biology*, 7: 33-53.

Soberon, F.; Lukas, J.L.; Van Amburgh, M.E.; Capuco, A.V.; Galton, D.M.; Overton, T.R., 2010. *J. Dairy Sci.*, 93: 556-573.

Sonier B, Arseneault M, Lavigne C, Ouellette, RJ and Vaillancourt C. The 5-HT2A serotoninergic receptor is expressed in the MCF-7 human breast cancer cell line and reveals a mitogenic effect of serotonin. *Biochemical and Biophysical Research Communications* 2006; 343(4): 1053-1059.

Spiegelman, B.M.; Flier, J.S., 2001. *Cell*, 104: 531-543.

Stanisiewski, R.A.; Erdman, L.W.; Douglass; Dahl, G.E., 1985. *J. Dairy Sci.*, 68: 1134-1140. http://classes.ansci.illinois.edu/ansc438/lactation/lactationresources.htm

Stelwagen, K., 2001. *J. Dairy Sci.*, 84 (Electronic supplement): E204-E211.

Stelwagen, K.; Phyn, C.V.C.; Davis, S.R.; Guinard-Flament, J.; Pomies, D.; Roche, J.R.; Kay, J.K. 2013. *J. Dairy Sci.*, 96(6): 3401–3413.

Stockdale, C.R., 2006. *Australian Journal of Experimental Agriculture*, 46: 965-974.

Strang, B.D.; Bertics, S.J.; Grummer, R.R.; Armentano, L.E., 1998. *J. Dairy Sci.*, 81: 728-739.

Strapakova, E.; Juraj, C.; Peter, S., 2016. *Arch. Anim. Breed.*, 59: 329-335; doi: 10.5194/aab-59: 329-2016.

Strucken, E.; Laurenson, Y.; Brockmann, G., 2015. *Front. Genet.*, 6: 118. Doi: 10.3389/fgene. 2015.00118

Stull MA, Pai V, Vomachka AJ, Marshall AM, Jacob GA and Horseman ND. Mammary gland homeostasis employs serotonergic regulation of epithelial tight junctions. *Proc. Natl. Acad. Sci. U.S.A.* 2007; 104.

Swan, H.; Broster, W., 1980. *J. Dairy Sci.*, 63: 1514-1529.

Takeshi, Y.; Hisato, T.; Akiko, N.; Youji, S.; Naoko, S.; Kenji, T., 2011. *J. Anim. Sci.*, 24(5): 610-615 doi: 10.5713/ajas.2011.10271.

Terao, H., 2010. *J. Anim. Vet. Adv.*, 9: 2333-2337.

Tiong, T.S.; Herington, A.C., 1991. *Endocrinol.*, 129: 1628-1634.

Torner, L.; Karg, S.; Blume A.; Kandasamy M.; Kuhn H.G.; Winkler, J.; Aigner, L.; Neumann, I.D.,2009. *J. Neurosci*, 29: 1826-33.

Trayhurn, P.; Gouglas, J.B.; McGuckin, M.M., 1982. Brown adipose tissue thermogenesis is suppressed during lactation in mice. *Nature,* 298: 59-69.

Tucker, H.A., 1981. *J. Dairy Sci.,* 64: 1403-1421.

Tucker, H.A., 1987. *J. Dairy Sci.,* 70: 1958-1966.

Umesh, Singh; Rajib, Deb; Rafeeque, Rahman Alyethodi; Rani, Alex; Sushil, Kumar; Sandip, Chakraborty; Kuldeep, Dhama; Arjava, Sharma, 2014. *Biomarkers and Genomic Medicine,* 6: 49-58.

Underwood, J.P.; Drackley, J.K.; Clark, J.H., 2001. *J. Dairy Sci.,* 84(Supply1): 364 (Abstr).

Urdaz, J.H.; Overton, M.W.; Moore, D.A.; Santos, J.E.P., 2006. *J. Dairy Sci.,* 89: 2000-2006. (www.omafra.gov.on.ca)

V.G. Smith, T.W. Beck, E.M. Convey, H.A. 1974. *Neuro endocrinology,* 15: 172-181.

V.G. Smith, T.W. Beck, E.M. Convey, H.A. Tucker.1974. *Neuro-endocrinology,* 15(3-4): 172-181.

Van Den Top, A.M.; Wensing, T.; Geelen, M.J.H.; Wentink, G.H.; Vant Klooster, A.T.; Beynen, A.C., 1995. *J. Dairy Sci.,* 78: 2208-2220.

Van Saun, R.J.; Idleman, S.C.; Sniffen, C.J., 1993. *J. Dairy Sci.,* 76: 236-244.

Vanoye-Carlo, A.; Morales, T.; Aguilar, E.; Mendoza Rodriguez, A.; Cerbon, M.A., 2008. *Horm Behav.,* 53: 112-113.

Velazquez-Villegas, L.A.; Tovar, A.R.; Lopez-Barradas, A.M.; Torres, N., 2013. *PLOS ONE* 8(7): e69338. doi:10.1371/journal.pone.0069338.

Vetharaniam, I.; Davis, S.R.; Soboleva, T.K.; Shorten, P.R.; Wake, G.C. 2003. *J. Dairy Sci.,* 86: 1987-1996.

Vicini, J.L.; Buonomo, F.C.; Veenhuizen, J.J.; Miller, M.A.; Clemmons, D.R.; Collier, R.J., 1991. *J. Nutr.,* 121: 1656-1664.

Vigneaud, D.U.; Ressler, B.; Swan, C.; Roberts, JM.; Katsoyannis, P.G., 1954. *J. Am. Chem. Soc.,* 76: 3115-3121.

Vilaro, S.; Vinas, O.; Remesar, X.; Herrera, E., 1987. *Pharmacology Biochem. & Behavior,* 27: 333-339.

Wall, E.H.; Crawford, H.M.; Ellis, S.E.; Dahl, G.E.; McFadden, T.B. 2006. *J. Dairy Sci.,* 89: 4640-4648.

Wall, E.H.; McFadden, T.B. 2008. *J. Ani. Sci.,* 86 (Supplement13): 27-36 (BOLFA supplement).

Wall, E.H.; McFadden, T.B., 2007. *J. Dairy Sci.,* 90: 5042-5048.

Wall, E.H.; McFadden, T.B., 2007. *J. Dairy Sci.,* 90: 716-720.

Wan, Y.; Lin, T.; Lain, J.; Chen, H.; Shyu, C., 1988. *Journal of Taiwan Livestock Research,* 31(1): 87-100.

Watters, J.J.; Swank, M.W.; Wilkinson, C.W.; Dorsa, D.M., 1996. *Peptides,* 17(1): 67-73.

Webb, R.; Garnsworthy, P.C.; Gong, J.G.; Armstrong, D.G., 2004. *J. Anim. Sci.,* 82 E-Suppl: E63-74.

Weigle, D.S.; Selfridge, L.E.; Schwartz, M.W.; Seeley, R.J.; Cummings, D.E.; Havel, P.J.; Kuijper, J.L.; BeltrandelRio, H., 1998. *Diabetes,* 47: 298-302.

Whittemore, C.T., 1980. *Lactation of the dairy cow.* Longman, New York.

Wilde CJ, Addey CVP, Boddy LM and Peaker M. Autocrine regulation of milk secretion by a protein in milk. *Biochemical Journal* 1995; 305: 51–58.

Wilde, C.J.; Knight, C.H.; Addey, C.V.P.; Blatchford, D.R.; Travers, M.; Bennett, C.N.; Peaker. M., 1990. *Protoplasma,* 159: 112-117, DOI: 10.1007/BF01322594.

Wilde, C.J.; Addey, C.V.P.; Boddy, L.M.; Peaker, M., 1995. *Biochemical Journal,* 305: 51-58.

Wilde, C.J.; Knight, C.H.; Addey, C.V.P.; Blatchford, D.R.; Travers, M.; Bennett, C.N.; Peaker, M., 1990. *Protoplasma,* 159: 112-117.

Wilde, C.J.; Peaker, M., 1990. *J. Agric. Sci.,* 114: 235-238.

Wilde, Caroline, C.J.V.P.; Peaker, M., 1996. *J. Physiol.,* 491(2): 465-469.

Williams, P.D.; Anderson, P.S.; Ball, R.G.; Bock, M.G.; Carroll, L.; Chiu, S.H.; Clineschmidt, B.V.; Culberson, J.C.; Erb, J.M.; Evans, B.E., 1994. *Journal of Med. Chem.,* 37(5): 565-71.

Williams, P.D.; Clineschmidt, B.V.; Erb, J.M.; Freidinger, R.M.; Guidotti, M.T.; Lis, E.V.; Pawluczyk, J.M.; Pettibone, D.J.; Reiss, D.R.; Veber, D.F., 1995. *J. Med. Chem.,* 38(23): 4634-4636.

Williams; G.L.; Gazal, O.S.; Leshin, L.S.; Stanko, R.L.; Anderson, L.L., 2001. *Biol. Reprod.,* 65: 295-300.

Woodword, T.L.; Xie, J.W.; Haslan, S.Z., 1998. *J. Mammary Gland Biol. & Neoplasia,* 3: 117-131.

Wyatt, P.G.; Allen, M.J.; Chilcott, J.; Foster, A.; Livermore, D.G.; Mordaunt, J.E.; Scicinski, J.; Woollard, P.M., 2002. *Bioorganic & Medicinal Chemistry Letters*, 12(10): 1399-404. http://en. wikipedia.org/wiki/Oxytocin_receptor.

Xiao, X.Q.; Grove, K.L.; Grayson, B.E.; Smith, M.S., 2004. *Endocrinology*, 145: 830-838.

Yadav, G. Roy, A.K. and Mahendra Singh.2015. *Indian J. Anim. Nutr.* 32(2): 133-138.

Yallowitz, A.R.; Alexandrova, E.M.; Talos, F.; Xu, S.; Marchenko, N.D.; Moll, U.M., 2014. *Cell Death Differ.*, 21(4): 645-54. doi: 10.1038/cdd.2013.199.

Zelena, D.; Makara, G.B.; Nagy, G.M.; 2003. *Endocrine*, 147-52.

Zhu, L.H.; Armentano, L.E.; Bremmer, D.R.; Grummer, R.R.; Bertics, S.J., 2000. *J. Dairy Sci.*, 83: 734-740.

Zieba, D.A.; Szczesna, M.; Klocek-Gorka, B.; Molik, E.; Misztal, T.; Williams, G.L.; Romanowicz, K.; Stepien, E.; Keisler, D.H.; Murawski, M., 2008. *Domestic Anim. Endocrinol.*, 34(2): 196-203.

□□□